A Word from One of Canada's Foremost Scientists

More Vitality Cooking *provides an excellent opportunity for Canadians to make a tangible investment in their personal health and that of their loved ones. We've known for a long time that the foods we eat can influence our risk of diseases such as cancer and heart disease. Studies have shown that populations who eat more fruits and vegetables are generally healthier.*

As well, we have learned over the past several years that health promotion and cancer prevention depend upon the interplay between our genetic heritage and our lifestyle, which includes the food we choose to eat.

More Vitality Cooking *is a sound and practical guide for a nutritious and delicious diet. I wholeheartedly recommend this book to anyone who wants a healthy lifestyle for themselves and their family.*

DR. ALAN BERNSTEIN

DIRECTOR, SAMUEL LUNENFELD RESEARCH INSTITUTE OF MOUNT SINAI HOSPITAL, TORONTO, ONTARIO

PROFESSOR, DEPARTMENT OF MOLECULAR AND MEDICAL GENETICS, UNIVERSITY OF TORONTO

Also by Monda Rosenberg and Frances Berkoff

The Vitality Cookbook

Praise for *The Vitality Cookbook*

"With today's trend toward personal management of health and
lifestyle, *The Vitality Cookbook* is right on the mark ...
above others in the field."

Quill & Quire

"The appealing recipes in *The Vitality Cookbook* make eating fruits
and vegetables a pleasure — and may even prolong
our lives in the bargain!"

Jacques Pépin

"Excellent ... abundant with fruits and vegetables ... nutrition-wise ...."

The Calgary Herald

"Healthy eating does not necessarily have to mean boring eating.
Case in point — *The Vitality Cookbook*."

The Canadian Jewish News

More Vitality Cooking

Full-Flavored, Easy Recipes Brimming with Fruits and Vegetables

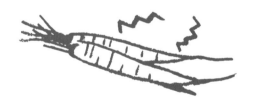

MONDA ROSENBERG
and FRANCES BERKOFF

A Lorraine Greey Book
HarperCollins*PublishersLtd*

The authors gratefully acknowledge a grant from the International Olive Oil Council

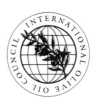

With Appreciation

A special thank you to all those who helped us, especially:
Anita Draycott, a superb editor, whose words added pizazz to our text. Dr. Venket Rao, Professor, Department of Nutritional Science, University of Toronto, for answering all our questions on phytochemicals and making sure our information was accurate. Holly Lee, who gave up weekends with her two adorable children to type our manuscript flawlessly. Andrea Emard, whose sharp eye once again caught all our mistakes. Marilyn Crowley and Trudy Patterson, the team that tested the Chatelaine recipes, who gave constant encouragement and sound advice. Barbara Dean, for cheerfully testing recipes and reading through our manuscript with her meticulous eye. Lucie Cousineau, for her infinite patience and support. Rona Maynard, who is always encouraging and supportive. Barbara Selley, for her expert nutritional analysis. Andrew Smith, for his imaginative design and calm manner. Joseph Gisini, for his brilliant way with the page layout. Ron Fiorelli, for his enthusiastic support. Jodi Macpherson, for her creative ideas and words of wisdom. Everyone at HarperCollins, for their commitment to this project. Lorraine Greey, for her expert guidance, enthusiasm and encouragement. Michael O'Neail, our professional recipe taster, who made us laugh.

First Edition

Canadian Cataloguing in Publication Data
Rosenberg, Monda
　More vitality cooking : full-flavored, easy recipes brimming with fruits and vegetables

"A Lorraine Greey book".
ISBN 0-00-638535-4

1. Cookery (Fruit).　2. Cookery (Vegetables).
3. Low-fat diet - Recipes.　I. Berkoff, Frances G.
II. Title.

TX714.R665 1997　641.6'4　C96-931880-4

97 98 99 00 01 02 ❖ WEB 10 9 8 7 6 5 4 3 2 1

Produced for HarperCollins Publishers Ltd
by Lorraine Greey Publications Ltd.
Suite 303, 56 The Esplanade
Toronto, Canada M5E 1A7

Design: Andrew Smith

Page layout and composition:
　Joseph Gisini, Andrew Smith Graphics, Inc.

Cover illustrations: Grant Innes

Other illustrations: Jeff Jackson/Reactor

Printed and bound in Canada

Contents

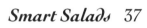

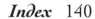

More Vitality

IMAGINE WALKING INTO A GROCERY STORE AND filling up your cart with items that could reduce your risk of developing heart disease or cancer, help you lose weight, maybe even slow down some of the health hazards of aging. No doubt these items would be on your regular grocery list!

What are these wonder foods? Fresh produce — pure and simple. More and more research indicates that a mix of fruits and vegetables eaten daily helps maintain good health throughout our lives.

Of course this isn't really news. But studies show that we're a bit slow to respond to nutritionists' recommendations to eat at least five, ideally ten, servings of these healthy, delicious foods every day.

WHY FRUITS AND VEGETABLES?

Fruits and vegetables contain fiber, vitamin C, folic acid, vitamin A and numerous minerals, including potassium, calcium and iron. They're also rich in compounds called phytochemicals ("phyto" is Greek for plant). These phytochemicals differ from vitamins and minerals in that they have no known nutritional value, but act in a variety of ways to offer front-line defense against disease. As well, most fruits and vegetables are almost fat-free.

Obesity and health problems are on the rise. Yet we're a nation that seems focused on low-fat foods. Our message: Instead of concentrating on cutting back, treat your body to the healthful benefits of fruits and vegetables.

Populations who eat more fruits and vegetables have less heart disease and less cancer and are generally healthier. All our recipes are chock-full of all the healthiest produce, and we've kept the fat and calories relatively low so you can indulge deliciously without guilt.

NATURE'S MEDICINE CHEST

A single carrot or wedge of cantaloupe contains a healthy amount of beta-carotene as well as hundreds of

FOLIC ACID

Recent studies link high blood levels of homocysteine, an amino acid, with an increased risk of heart disease. Folic acid appears to help lower homocysteine levels, thus lowering heart disease risk.

Folic acid is a key nutrient for women planning to get pregnant. This B vitamin is associated with reducing the risk of Neural Tube Defects that occur within the first month of conception. (Spina bifida is one of the more common defects.) Since the problem occurs when the fetus is about four weeks old, when most women aren't aware they are pregnant, it's important to get enough folic acid before you conceive.

The best food sources are dark-green leafy vegetables, spinach, orange juice, liver, peas, broccoli, brussels sprouts, asparagus, dried beans and lentils.

phytochemicals. Research has long shown that a diet rich in fruits and vegetables that are high in beta-carotene helps provide protection against heart disease and certain types of cancer. Results of a recent long-term study, however, in which healthy individuals took beta-carotene supplements, showed that pills alone provided no protection. So beta-carotene in isolation is not effective — but beta-carotene in its natural state in food is never on its own — it always keeps company with other members of the carotenoid family (a large family numbering up to 500) as well as other plant chemicals. It's believed that in the plant cells, they all work together to provide protection against compounds that could destroy the plant, and once they're in our system they protect our cells in a similar way. Just remember it's nature's natural mix of vitamins, minerals, phytochemicals and fiber — a whole slew of players, not a single chemical — that creates the best disease-fighting team. And it will be years, probably decades, before this complex mix and interaction of chemicals can be identified and reproduced in pill form. So remember, when you take that bite of broccoli, not only does it taste better than a pill but it's the best way we currently know of to have a disease-fighting patrol working for us.

Indulge and enjoy!

MONDA ROSENBERG AND FRANCES BERKOFF

NUTRIENT ANALYSIS

Nutrient analysis of recipes was done by Info Access (1988) Inc., Don Mills, Ontario, using the nutritional accounting component of the CBORD Menu Management System.

The nutrient database was the 1991 Canadian Nutrient File, supplemented with documented data from reliable sources.

Analysis is based on imperial weights and measures, the larger number of servings (i.e., smaller portion) and smaller ingredient quantity when there is a range, and the first ingredient listed when there is a choice. Optional ingredients and garnishes in unspecified amounts are not included.

Nutrient Information On Recipes: Nutrient values have been rounded to nearest whole number. Good and excellent sources of vitamins A and C, folacin, calcium and iron have been identified according to criteria established for nutrition labeling (Guide to Food Labelling and Advertising, 1996). A serving supplying 15% of Recommended Daily Intake (RDI) of a vitamin or mineral (30% for vitamin C) is a good source of that nutrient. An excellent source must supply 25% of the RDI (50% for vitamin C).

THE POWER OF PHYTOCHEMICALS

Phytochemicals in plants have physiological properties that can influence disease — cancer, heart disease, diabetes and other degenerative conditions — and help maintain good health. They work in many different ways and combinations: some, like antioxidants, protect against harmful cell damage; others stimulate the immune system or suppress growth of cancer cells; and others reduce the harmful effects of hormones such as estrogen.

Scientists are deciphering the many ways these chemicals in food offer frontline defense against disease. The major players include:

CAROTENOIDS

There are more than 500 different carotenoids, including beta-carotene, lycopene, alpha-carotene and lutein. These antioxidant plant pigments and free radical scavengers are found in dark-green vegetables such as spinach and broccoli, and orange-yellow fruits and vegetables such as cantaloupe, carrots, sweet potatoes and apricots.

Lycopene, the red pigment in tomatoes, is the most potent carotenoid. It has been shown to lower risk of cancer and heart disease.

MONOTERPENES

The aromatic compounds that give flavor to citrus fruits and herbs such as dill, caraway and mint inhibit certain tumor growth.

PHYTOSTEROLS

Plant sterols that compete with cholesterol for absorption and may also be anti-carcinogenic, phytosterols are found in soy beans, sesame seeds, sesame oil and legumes.

SAPONINS

The bitter compounds present in cruciferous vegetables such as broccoli, brussels sprouts, cabbage, cauliflower and turnip, as well as beans, chickpeas and soy beans can help lower cholesterol levels and act as immune stimulators and anti-carcinogens.

PHYTOESTROGENS

These plant hormones may block the activity of estrogen on cancer cells. They are found in legumes such as soy beans, lentils and oats, and in high levels in flax.

ISOFLAVONOIDS

Found in soy beans, lentils and licorice, this family of compounds is thought to influence hormone-related diseases such as breast and prostate cancers.

FLAVONOIDS

These potent antioxidants are being studied for their anti-inflammatory and anti-cancer properties. Anthocyanin, the pigment present in strawberries, blueberries, raspberries and grapes, is particularly beneficial.

ALLYL SULFIDES

Found in garlic and onions, they help control blood pressure, lower risk of heart disease, stimulate the immune system and may help the body get rid of cancer-causing substances.

POLYPHENOL FLAVONOIDS

Found in tea (green and black) and herbs such as oregano and sage, they are being studied for their anti-cancer activity.

Light Bites and Little Courses

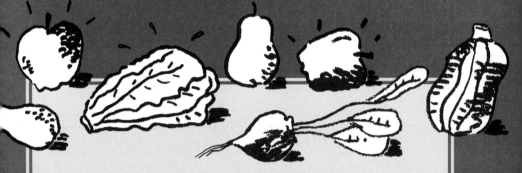

Moroccan Grilled Eggplant Dip

Light 'n' Lemony Smoked Salmon Dip

Quesadillas with Ripe Mango, Chèvre and Coriander

Southwestern Scallops with Garlic and Hot Peppers

Shrimp and Mango Bruschetta

Smoked Chicken Rolls with Light Lime Cream

Best-Ever Shrimp Appetizer

Grilled Shrimp with Roasted Red Pepper Sauce

Mimi's Mussels Rockefeller

Moroccan Grilled Eggplant Dip

Roasted vegetables are blended into a robust, low-cal dip — so nudge out predictable high-fat appetizers and save your appetite for the main course.

PREPARATION TIME: 15 MINUTES / GRILLING TIME: 20 MINUTES
STANDING TIME: 30 MINUTES / MAKES: 3½ CUPS

1 large eggplant
1 large or 2 small onions
4 large plum or 2 regular tomatoes
2 tbsp olive oil
1 to 2 crushed garlic cloves
1 lemon
¼ cup chopped fresh parsley
1 tsp ground cumin
½ tsp salt
¼ tsp freshly ground black pepper

1. Preheat barbecue and lightly oil grill. Cut unpeeled eggplant lengthwise into ½-inch slices. Cut onion crosswise into 1-inch slices. (If onions are small, slice in half.) Halve tomatoes lengthwise. Stir oil with garlic.

2. Brush cut vegetables with garlic oil. Place on barbecue and grill, turning often, until eggplant and tomatoes are slightly charred and onion is tender, about 10 to 15 minutes for eggplant and tomatoes, and 20 minutes for onion. Remove vegetables from grill as they are done. Meanwhile, squeeze juice from lemon.

3. Finely chop grilled vegetables using a large knife, or by whirling in a food processor using an on-and-off motion. Place in a mixing bowl and stir in 3 tablespoons lemon juice, parsley, cumin, salt and pepper. Let stand at room temperature for at least 30 minutes to develop flavors. Taste and add more lemon juice and seasonings, if you wish. Dip can be stored, covered, in the refrigerator for up to 3 days. Bring to room temperature and serve with vegetable crudités or pita triangles.

PER TABLESPOON

Calories: 9

Protein: Trace

Fat: 1 g

Carbohydrate: 1 g

Fiber: Trace

Light 'n' Lemony Smoked Salmon Dip

Toronto caterer Sandra Watson cleverly used light sour cream to create this superb smoked salmon dip. The cheaper smoked salmon ends or bits work just as well as the expensive thin slices.

PREPARATION TIME: 15 MINUTES / COOKING TIME: 30 SECONDS
REFRIGERATION TIME: 1 HOUR
MAKES: 2 CUPS DIP, ABOUT 8 SERVINGS

½ lb (250 g) smoked salmon
1 cup light or regular sour cream
1 tbsp drained capers
1 tbsp chopped fresh dill
1½ tsp lemon juice
Dash of hot pepper sauce
1½ lbs (750 g) sugar snap peas or snow peas, or slices of sweet pepper

1. In a food processor, chop smoked salmon using an on-and-off motion. Add remaining ingredients except peas and whirl until almost smooth. Taste, and add more lemon juice or hot pepper sauce, if you like. Turn mixture into a serving dish. Use right away or cover with plastic wrap and refrigerate until cold, about 1 hour or up to 1 day.

2. If using peas, trim off ends. Half fill a large saucepan with water. Bring to a full rolling boil over high heat. Meanwhile, place a colander in the sink. When water is boiling rapidly, add peas all at once. As soon as peas are bright green, about 30 to 45 seconds, remove from heat. Pour them into colander and drain. Rinse peas with cold running water until they are cool. Drain well. Cover peas and refrigerate until dip is cold.

3. Serve dip on a large plate surrounded by peas or peppers for dipping. To take on a picnic, spoon a little dip into plastic glasses and stand peas, with their ends in the dip, around edge of glass. Cover with plastic wrap.

SUGAR SNAP PEAS

About as long as your baby finger, crisp sweet sugar snap peas are a cross between traditional garden peas and flat snow peas. You can eat their fat rounded pods — peas, shell and all — except for the stem! Serve them raw with dips or on a relish tray. Lightly steamed, sugar snap peas need little adornment since their sweet garden-fresh flavor is outstanding. Try adding slivers of sugar snap peas at the last minute to stir-fries, soups and risottos for a crisp texture contrast.

PER SERVING

Calories:	100
Protein:	10 g
Fat:	3 g
Carbohydrate:	9 g
Fiber:	2 g
Excellent source:	Vitamin C

Quesadillas with Ripe Mango, Chèvre and Coriander

A warm tortilla wedge oozing mango and peppery chèvre is one of the fastest, classiest canapés you can make. Add strips of red pepper for the holidays. In the summer, grill the quesadillas on the barbie.

PREPARATION TIME: 5 MINUTES / COOKING TIME: 8 MINUTES
MAKES: 16 APPETIZERS

PER APPETIZER

Calories: 36

Protein: 1 g

Fat: 1 g

Carbohydrate: 6 g

Fibre: Trace

1 very ripe mango
½ cup fresh coriander leaves
2 large (10-inch) tortillas or 4 small (6-inch) tortillas
2 tbsp creamy chèvre
Coarsely ground black pepper
Pinch of cayenne pepper
½ tsp olive oil or butter

QUICK QUESADILLAS

A quesadilla (kay-sa-dee-a) is a pronto Tex-Mex version of a grilled-cheese sandwich. Not your average snack food, it packs protein in every bite. Simply sprinkle a yummy filling like grated Monterey Jack cheese and sliced green onions over half a large flour tortilla. Fold and flip into a hot frying pan. Cook over medium heat until golden and the cheese begins to ooze, about 1 to 2 minutes per side. Cut into wedges for a satisfying appetizer, or add soup or a salad and you've got supper. Each of our filling suggestions is enough for one large tortilla. Olé!

HOW TO QUESADILLA

Lay a large (10-inch) flour tortilla flat on the counter. Cover half with filling, then fold the uncovered side over filling. Set a large frying pan over medium heat. Put the folded tortilla in the hot pan and cook until golden, about 2 minutes per side. Slice into 3 or 4 wedges.

MARIACHI

Sprinkle half the tortilla with 2 tablespoons well-drained, finely chopped seeded tomatoes or spread with 2 tablespoons salsa. Sprinkle with ½ cup grated cheddar or Monterey Jack cheese and 2 tablespoons chopped fresh coriander or thinly sliced green onions.

1. Peel mango. Thinly slice pulp from the stone. Wash and dry coriander leaves. Lay tortillas on the counter. Thinly spread chèvre over each tortilla, covering it right to edges. Add a generous grinding of black pepper, then a sprinkle of cayenne.

2. Cover half of each tortilla with thin mango slices. Scatter coriander over top. Lift up the uncovered side and fold it over filling. Lightly brush both sides of folded tortilla with oil.

3. Set a large frying pan over medium heat. Pick up folded tortilla by grasping the open edges at opposite sides and supporting the tortilla with your fingers. Place it in the hot pan. Cook until golden, about 2 minutes per side. Remove to a cutting board. Repeat with remaining tortilla. Immediately slice each into 8 wedges and serve hot. They look great arranged on a single dinner plate with a cluster of coriander in the center.

WINTER FRUIT HORS D'OEUVRES

Simply stir together 2 peeled diced kiwi, 1 cup chopped strawberries, a 10-oz (284-mL) can drained chopped mandarin oranges, 1 teaspoon lemon juice, ½ teaspoon brown sugar and 1 teaspoon finely chopped crystallized ginger in syrup. Serve a bowl of this festive salsa with Brie or mascarpone cheese and crisp crackers, or spread baguette slices with chèvre and spoon a little salsa on top. This salsa is also great spooned over ice cream or swirled in yogurt. *Makes 2 cups.*

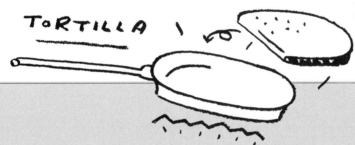

TORTILLA

CREAMY CHÈVRE

Lightly spread half the tortilla with 2 to 3 tablespoons creamy chèvre. Sprinkle with 2 tablespoons thinly sliced green onions and 2 tablespoons chopped well-drained tomatoes or chopped avocado. Top with a grinding of black pepper.

HAM AND SWISS

Sprinkle half the tortilla with ½ cup grated Swiss cheese and 1 slice of ham, cut into strips. Cover with torn pieces of spinach or romaine lettuce.

ANTIPASTO

Spread half the tortilla with ¼ cup antipasto, then sprinkle with 2 tablespoons grated Parmesan cheese.

BRIE AND STRAWBERRY

Thinly slice ripe Brie or Camembert. Thinly spread half the tortilla with 2 tablespoons strawberry jam. Lay strips of Brie on top.

TROPICAL

Thinly spread half the tortilla with 2 tablespoons light cream cheese. Top with ¼ cup chopped mango or papaya, then sprinkle with 2 tablespoons toasted coconut.

Southwestern Scallops with Garlic and Hot Peppers

When you're pressed for time but want to create a knockout first course or light dinner, buy small bay scallops (they're cheaper and sweeter than the large ones) and sauté in a buttery-tasting hot sauce. Spoon over couscous or rice or toss with fettuccine. Despite the indulgent taste, it's really low in fat.

PREPARATION TIME: 10 MINUTES / COOKING TIME: 10 MINUTES

MAKES: 3 TO 4 APPETIZER SERVINGS

PER SERVING

Calories: 106	
Protein: 15 g	
Fat: 2 g	
Carbohydrate: 5 g	
Fiber: 1 g	
Excellent source: Vitamin C	
Good source: Vitamin A	

1 small hot pepper, or 1 to 2 tbsp canned diced jalapeños

½ cup white wine

4 crushed garlic cloves

1 sweet red pepper

12 oz (375 g) bay scallops

1 tsp butter

Pinch of salt and white pepper

1 lime

SMART-BUY SCALLOPS

- Small bay scallops usually cost about half as much as shrimp and often less than salmon steaks. Resembling tiny marshmallows, bay scallops have a sweet fresh seafood taste and are more tender and succulent than the larger sea scallops.

- Bay scallops come from inshore and shallow offshore waters; the larger sea scallops grow in deeper offshore waters. The increased cost of harvesting sea scallops partially explains why they can cost twice as much as smaller bay scallops.

- A pound (500 g) of bay scallops nets about 40 small scallops; a pound of sea scallops averages about 18. So for pasta sauces and stir-fries, bay scallops yield more bites for your dollar.

- If you're calorie counting, a 3-ounce (100-g) scallop serving (before cooking) has 14 g of protein, only 75 calories and less than 1 g of fat.

- The best news is for the cholesterol-conscious: unlike shrimp and lobster, scallops contain very little cholesterol.

1. Seed fresh hot pepper and finely dice. Put hot pepper in a medium-size frying pan along with wine and garlic. Set pan over medium heat. Boil mixture gently, stirring often, for 5 minutes.

2. Meanwhile, seed red pepper and slice into thin bite-size pieces. Rinse scallops with cold water and drain. Do not pat them dry.

3. When garlic mixture has simmered for 5 minutes, add red pepper, scallops and butter. Turn heat to medium-high and stir-fry until scallops are opaque, about 2 to 3 minutes. Add salt and white pepper to taste. Squeeze juice from half a lime over top.

Shrimp and Mango Bruschetta

This clever, elegant appetizer comes from Kevin MacKeachie, a talented young Toronto chef. It's impressive whether it's served at a pool party, backyard wedding or Christmas cocktail affair. It doesn't require baking, cooking or pastry rolling.

PREPARATION TIME: 30 MINUTES / STANDING TIME: 30 MINUTES

MAKES: 6 CUPS SALSA, ENOUGH FOR 24 APPETIZERS

1 large ripe mango
1½-inch piece fresh ginger
2 to 3 limes
½ tsp salt
2 tbsp olive oil
1 large red pepper, seeded
1 small red onion
4 green onions
12 to 16 oz (375 to 500 g) cooked baby shrimp, the smaller the better
1 large ripe avocado (optional)
2 thin baguettes
Chopped coriander

PER APPETIZER

Calories: 50

Protein: 3 g

Fat: 1 g

Carbohydrate: 7 g

Fiber: Trace

Good source: Vitamin C

1. Peel the mango and cut the fruit away from stone. Finely slice about two-thirds of the mango pulp into a small dice, so pieces are about ¼ inch wide. Put diced mango in a large bowl.

2. Place remaining mango in a food processor. Peel fresh ginger. Coarsely chop the ginger and add it to mango in the food processor. Squeeze juice from limes and add 6 tablespoons of juice to the mango and ginger mixture. Add salt. Whirl, using an on-and-off motion until ginger is minced. Stop to scrape down sides occasionally. Whirl and gradually add oil through feed tube. Pour this mixture over chopped mango and stir until coated.

3. Finely chop red pepper and onion. Thinly slice green onions. Stir into mango mixture.

4. If shrimp are frozen, place them in a sieve and run cold tap water over them until all ice crystals disappear. Drain well. Pat dry with paper towels. If shrimp are not tiny, coarsely chop and stir into salsa.

5. Peel avocado. Dice and stir into salsa. Let it stand at room temperature for 30 minutes or in refrigerator for several hours. Slice baguette into rounds. Spoon mixture onto baguette slices and sprinkle with coriander. Or spoon into store-bought cocktail-size pastry cups or a glass bowl set in the center of a large platter. Always sprinkle with chopped coriander. Surround the bowl with pieces of endive to spoon salsa into, leafy lettuce leaves to roll around the salsa, small pitas to fill with salsa or crackers for dipping or topping with salsa. For an intriguing first course, serve on a bed of greens.

MAKE AHEAD: *The flavor will be better if this salsa is made a day before serving, then refrigerated. Wait until just before serving, however, to add avocado and shrimp, because avocado will darken and shrimp will soften.*

Smoked Chicken Rolls with Light Lime Cream

Simply roll up a tortilla filled with healthy ingredients, then slice into colorful rounds for a new sophisticated take on rolled party sandwiches.

PREPARATION TIME: 10 MINUTES / REFRIGERATION TIME: 1 HOUR

MAKES: 36 ROUNDS

8 oz (250 g) sliced smoked chicken or turkey

1 ripe avocado, peeled (optional)

3 carrots

1 lime

½ cup light sour cream

¼ tsp hot pepper sauce

6 small (6-inch) flour tortillas

¼ cup chopped fresh coriander or thinly sliced green onions

Shredded lettuce or fresh spinach (optional)

1. Slice chicken into ¼-inch bite-size strips. Cut avocado, if using, into slices. Cut carrots into thin strips. Grate peel from lime and stir into sour cream along with hot pepper sauce.

2. To assemble, lay tortillas flat. Thinly spread each tortilla with sour cream mixture. Place chicken strips in a line across middle of each tortilla. Top with carrot and avocado. Dab with any remaining sour cream mixture. Sprinkle with coriander or green onions. Top with a little lettuce, if you wish. Roll each into a cigar shape. Wrap each roll in waxed paper or plastic wrap and twist ends. Refrigerate at least until cold or for up to half a day. Slice into 1-inch rounds before serving.

APPETIZER ROLL-UP

Spread a 4½-oz (140-g) package herbed chèvre over 3 large tortillas. Lay fresh basil leaves in a strip across the center. Place a row of drained hot pickled peppers or pimiento strips or your favorite julienned vegetables such as peppers, carrots or zucchini beside basil. Roll up snugly. Wrap tightly in waxed paper or plastic wrap and twist ends. Refrigerate at least until chilled. Slice into 1-inch rounds. *Makes 24 appetizers.*

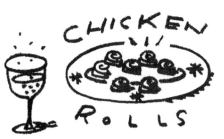

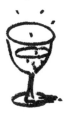

PER ROUND

Calories: 33	
Protein: 2 g	
Fat: 1 g	
Carbohydrate: 4 g	
Fiber: Trace	
Good source: Vitamin A	

Best-Ever Shrimp Appetizer

Voted the best shrimp appetizer we've ever made, this is the starter we love to make for any party special enough to splurge on shrimp. Buy cooked zipper-back shrimp with the tails on, toss with the marinade and you've got an unbelievably good appetizer in 5 minutes. The inexpensive papaya stretches the shrimp and adds a passion fruit taste.

PREPARATION TIME: 5 MINUTES / REFRIGERATION TIME: 1 HOUR
MAKES: 6 TO 8 SERVINGS, ABOUT 40 SHRIMPS

2 limes
2-inch piece of fresh ginger, or 1 tbsp bottled minced ginger
2 large garlic cloves, crushed
1 tbsp olive oil
1 tbsp soy or teriyaki sauce
1 tsp sugar
½ tsp hot red pepper flakes
½ small bunch fresh coriander
1½ to 2 lbs (750 g to 1 kg) large shrimp, cooked and frozen or fresh
2 to 3 ripe papayas

1. Squeeze limes and pour ¼ cup juice into a small dish. If using fresh ginger, remove peel. Grate on a ginger grater, or finely grind in a mini grinder, or finely chop and press through a garlic press. Stir ginger into lime juice along with garlic, oil, soy sauce, sugar and red pepper flakes. Coarsely chop enough coriander to measure ½ cup and set aside.

2. If using frozen cooked shrimp, simply place them in a large sieve. Run cold water over them until all ice crystals are melted. If shells are on, remove them if you like but leave tails on. Then, place in a bowl.

PAPAYA

One medium-size papaya contains 122 calories, but it's heavy with nutrients. It contains three times our recommended dietary allowance for vitamin C, calcium, and small amounts of the B vitamins, iron and zinc. It is also an excellent source of potassium. Papayas are actually large berries, good eaten fresh or cooked, wonderful in a fruit salad or salsa or as an accompaniment to seafood and chicken.

PER SERVING

Calories: 178

Protein: 25 g

Fat: 4 g

Carbohydrate: 11 g

Fiber: 2 g

Excellent source: Vitamin C

Good source: Vitamin A, Iron

3. Or, cook fresh shrimp in boiling water, covered, until all shrimp are bright pink and firm, about 2 minutes. Immediately drain into a large sieve. Run cold water over shrimp to quickly chill. Shell and place in a bowl.

4. Whisk the soy sauce mixture. Stir in shrimp, then chopped coriander. Refrigerate. Peel papayas and slice in half lengthwise. Scoop out black seeds and discard. Cut pulp into bite-size pieces. Stir into shrimp mixture. Keep refrigerated at least 1 hour or for up to 4 hours. If refrigerating longer, drain off marinade or it will overpower the delicate shrimp taste.

5. Serve in a shallow dish such as a large quiche dish, sprinkled liberally with fresh coriander leaves. Serve with toothpicks and lots of napkins or give guests small plates to spoon shrimp and papaya onto.

SHRIMP, MANGO AND RED PEPPER SALAD: *For an elegant starter prepare shrimp as above omitting papaya. Just before serving, slice 1 large mango and 1 large red pepper into small strips. Stir into shrimp mixture. Serve on a bed of mixed greens such as Boston lettuce, arugula and curly endive.*

Grilled Shrimp with Roasted Red Pepper Sauce

Dip juicy, plump, grilled shrimp, flavored with orange and a touch of cayenne, into a smoky, roasted red pepper sauce.

PREPARATION TIME: 30 MINUTES / BARBECUING TIME: 30 MINUTES

MAKES: 6 SERVINGS

SAUCE
4 red peppers
1 crushed garlic clove
2 tsp balsamic vinegar
½ tsp salt
Pinch of cayenne pepper (optional)
2 tbsp chopped Italian parsley or coriander

NEW-WAVE COCKTAIL SAUCE

Using a food processor fitted with a metal blade, drop 1 crushed garlic clove, ¼ cup fresh basil leaves or 1 teaspoon dried basil through feed tube while motor is running. Whirl, using an on-and-off motion, for about 10 seconds. Add 19-oz (540-mL) can drained tomatoes. Continue whirling, using an on-and-off motion, until mixture is chunky. Taste and add salt and cayenne as needed. Stir in ½ teaspoon horseradish and refrigerate up to 2 days. *Makes 2 cups.*

PER SERVING

Calories: 173	
Protein: 24 g	
Fat: 4 g	
Carbohydrate: 9 g	
Fiber: 2 g	
Excellent source: Vitamin A, Vitamin C	
Good source: Iron	

SHRIMP

2 lbs (1 kg) large raw shrimp, with or without shells, fresh or frozen (see below)*

¼ cup undiluted frozen orange juice concentrate

2 tbsp olive oil

2 crushed garlic cloves

½ tsp salt

¼ tsp cayenne pepper

2 tbsp chopped fresh parsley or coriander (optional)

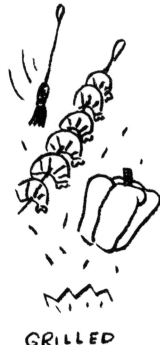

1. Preheat barbecue or broiler. Oil grill or coat broiling pan with cooking spray. Grill whole peppers, turning often, until they are blistered on all sides, about 25 to 30 minutes. Place blackened peppers in a paper bag. Seal and let sit until peppers are cool enough to handle, about 10 minutes. Peel away skin, then core and seed peppers, saving juices. In a food processor, whirl peppers and juice with garlic, vinegar and salt. For a fiery taste, add cayenne. Whirl until almost smooth. Stir in parsley. Use right away or store, covered, in the refrigerator for up to 3 days, or freeze. Bring to room temperature before serving.

2. If shrimp are frozen, run them under cold water until ice crystals disappear. Thread shrimp onto skewers. Stir orange juice with oil, garlic, salt and cayenne. Generously brush over shrimp. Grill, brushing often with orange juice mixture, until shrimp are bright pink and hot, about 2 minutes per side. (If making ahead, grill the shrimp, immediately refrigerate for up to half a day and serve cold.) Serve sprinkled with chopped parsley, with roasted pepper sauce for dipping. This sauce is also wonderful over fish steaks.

GRILLED SHRIMP

JUICY SHRIMP: Grill shrimp with shells on. When purchasing frozen shrimp, look for bags marked "zipper-back" for easy peeling. Let guests peel their own grilled shrimp before dipping in red pepper sauce. If you remove shell before grilling, leave tail attached both for good looks and as a handy holder when eating.

Mimi's Mussels Rockefeller

These juicy mussels, cooked up by Mimi Findlay, owner of Mimi's Ocean Grill in Mahone Bay, N.S., nestle in their shells with a garlicky spinach filling and a crisp crumb coating — perfect as a canapé. Inexpensive, they can be made ahead of time in big party batches and baked right out of the freezer.

PREPARATION TIME: 1 HOUR / STEAMING TIME: 10 MINUTES

BAKING TIME: 10 MINUTES / MAKES: 70 APPETIZERS

2½ lbs (1.25 kg) fresh mussels (about 70)

FILLING

10-oz (300-g) pkg frozen spinach, defrosted, or 1 bag or 2 bunches of fresh spinach

4-oz (125-g) pkg light cream cheese, about ½ cup, at room temperature

½ cup freshly grated Parmesan cheese

1 large crushed garlic clove

2 green onions, finely chopped

1 tbsp sherry or licorice-flavored liqueur (optional)

¼ tsp each of salt, freshly ground black pepper and hot pepper sauce

TOPPING

2 slices bread, or 1 cup fresh bread crumbs

2 tbsp finely chopped fresh parsley

1 tbsp melted butter or olive oil

1. Scrub mussels under cool running water and remove any beards. Discard any mussels that are open and will not close when gently tapped. Pour 1 inch water into a large saucepan, then add mussels. Cover pan and place over medium-high heat. Steam until mussels are opened, about 7 but no more than 9 minutes. Discard any mussels that do not open. Remove from heat and drain.

JODI'S CHEATER MUSSELS

Jodi MacPherson, a busy mother of three and great cook, discovered this instant wine mix that produces a superb Friday night dinner. Simply heat together an equal amount of white wine and hot salsa sauce — about ¼ to ⅓ cup of each works well. When bubbling, add 3 to 4 lbs (1.5 to 2 kg) scrubbed mussels. Cover, and simmer until mussels open, about 5 to 6 minutes. Stir occasionally. Place mussels in bowls and pour sauce over top. *Serves 2.*

PER MUSSEL

Calories:	16
Protein:	1 g
Fat:	1 g
Carbohydrate:	1 g
Fiber:	Trace

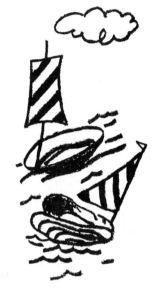

2. When mussels are cool enough to handle, remove them from their shells. Break half of the shells, the largest ones, into halves and place on shallow-sided baking sheets. Put 1 mussel in each shell. Refrigerate, uncovered, while continuing with recipe.

3. To make filling, squeeze defrosted frozen spinach between your hands to remove as much moisture as possible. Or wash fresh spinach under cold running water and remove stems; cook in the microwave or in a saucepan, stirring just until wilted, then drain and cool. When spinach is cool enough to handle, squeeze it firmly to remove as much moisture as possible. You should have about 1 cup spinach. Finely chop spinach. In a large mixing bowl, stir cream cheese with Parmesan, garlic, green onions, sherry, seasonings and hot pepper sauce until well blended. Then, stir in spinach.

4. To make topping, whirl bread in a food processor. Measure out 1 cup crumbs. Stir in parsley and butter.

5. Preheat oven to 375°F (190°C). Place a rounded teaspoon of the spinach mixture on top of each mussel. Spread spinach over mussels with your finger. Sprinkle each mussel with topping, patting down slightly. Bake in center of oven until hot and topping is golden, about 10 to 12 minutes. Serve right away.

MAKE AHEAD: *Assemble appetizers. Do not bake. Tightly cover with plastic wrap and refrigerate for up to 1 day or overwrap with foil and freeze for up to 1 month. Unwrap cold or frozen mussels. Do not defrost. Immediately place in a preheated 375°F (190°C) oven until hot and topping is golden, about 12 to 15 minutes.*

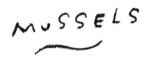

BUDGET MUSSELS

Mussels top the list of best buys in the seafood department.

- Sizing them up nutritionally, 1 pound (500 g) of mussels, about 35 in the shell, supplies 16 g of protein, 3 g of fat and 113 calories. They are also an excellent source of iron, providing 37% of our recommended daily intake.

- A pound (500 g) of mussels sells for $3 or less. Considering that a pound usually contains at least 35 mussels, one mussel costs less than a dime or about a tenth the price of a single oyster.

- Unlike shrimp, mussels travel well so we can buy fresh mussels any time of the year even in the middle of the Prairies.

Soups for All Occasions

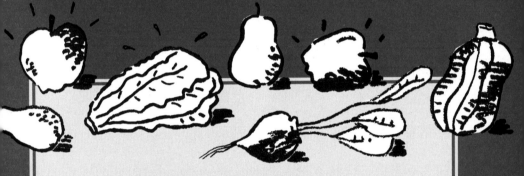

Sweet Potato and Mango Soup

Cool Cucumber-Yogurt Soup

Dilled Squash Soup

Curried Harvest Pumpkin Soup

Rona's Roasted Tomato Soup

Spring Chicken and Asparagus Soup

Two-Tone Melon Soup

Bloody Mary Soup with Vodka

Roasted Red Pepper Soup

Getaway Caribbean Chowder

Quick Curried Lentil and Carrot Soup

Sweet Potato and Mango Soup

Sounds divine, doesn't it? That's just why we ordered it at the 7 West Café on Charles St. in Toronto. Chef Robert MacDonald's approach in keeping the flavors pure and full did not disappoint. Superb before a big festive dinner or chilled before a barbecue fest.

PREPARATION TIME: 20 MINUTES / COOKING TIME: 30 MINUTES
MAKES: 14 ONE-CUP SERVINGS

1 large onion
2 tsp olive oil
4 large sweet potatoes, about 2 lbs (1 kg)
1 tsp curry powder
8 cups chicken broth or water
2 carrots
2 celery stalks, including leaves
2 large ripe mangoes
2 tbsp maple syrup (optional)

1. Coarsely chop onion. Heat oil in a large saucepan. Add onion and sauté, stirring often, over medium-low heat until soft, about 5 minutes.

2. Meanwhile, peel sweet potatoes and cut each into 6 to 8 pieces. When onions are soft, stir curry powder into onions. Increase heat to high. Add the broth or water. If adding water, stir in ½ teaspoon salt. Add potatoes. Cover and bring to a boil.

3. Meanwhile, peel carrots. Slice carrots and celery into ½-inch pieces and add to soup as soon as they are cut. When soup is boiling, decrease heat to medium-low and boil gently, covered, until vegetables are very soft, at least 20 and up to 40 minutes.

4. Meanwhile, peel mangoes. Slice pulp from stone. When potatoes and carrots are very soft, remove soup from heat. Pour most of liquid into a bowl. Put a portion of cooked vegetables into a food processor fitted with a metal blade along with about ¼ to ½ cup of liquid.

SASSY SPICY GAZPACHO

Coarsely chop 1 seeded green pepper, 1 small seeded English cucumber, 1 onion and 2 garlic cloves. Put in food processor fitted with a metal blade. Add 28-oz (796-mL) can plum tomatoes, including juice, 1 cup vegetable cocktail juice or spicy vegetable cocktail juice, 3 tablespoons red-wine vinegar, 3 tablespoons olive oil, 1 teaspoon cumin and ¼ teaspoon cayenne pepper. Whirl, using an on-and-off motion, until no large pieces remain. Refrigerate at least until cold or up to 1 day. *Makes 4 cups.*

PER SERVING

Calories:	110
Protein:	4 g
Fat:	2 g
Carbohydrate:	20 g
Fibre:	3 g
Excellent source:	Vitamin A
Good source:	Vitamin C

5. Purée, using an on-and-off motion, until mixture is fairly smooth. Add to soup broth. Repeat with remaining vegetables, adding mango pulp to last batch.

6. Taste soup, and stir in maple syrup, if you wish, 1 tablespoon at a time until as sweet as you like. Thin if necessary by stirring in water. Add salt if needed. Serve right away or refrigerate up to 3 days or freeze. Lovely served piping hot or cold with a swirl of yogurt and red pepper purée in the center or a swirl of pesto. A scattering of fresh coriander leaves is also nice.

MANGOES

Juicy, sweet mangoes are high in beta-carotene, vitamin C and fiber, and a whole mango has only 135 calories. Slice over your breakfast cereal, make a fresh mango salad for lunch, serve a mango salsa with fish or chicken or enjoy alone as a sweet, juicy snack.

Cool Cucumber-Yogurt Soup

Jalapeño peppers add pizazz to this refreshing summer soup. It was first served to us by Barbara Dean, a busy mother, who stocks it in her fridge in the summer for sipping around the pool.

PREPARATION TIME: 10 MINUTES / MAKES: 8 HALF-CUP SERVINGS

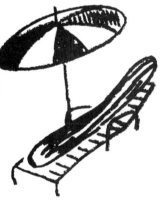

2 jalapeños or 1 banana pepper, seeded
1 crushed garlic clove
1 large English cucumber
2 green onions
¼ cup packed fresh parsley or coriander leaves
1 tbsp olive oil
¼ tsp salt
½ cup cold water, or 4 ice cubes
2 cups plain yogurt

1. Put jalapeño peppers and garlic in the bowl of a food processor. Whirl them until they are finely chopped. Coarsely slice unpeeled cucumber and green onions. Add to peppers along with parsley, oil and salt. Whirl until finely chopped but not puréed. Add water or ice cubes and whirl. Pour soup into a large bowl or refrigerator container. Stir in yogurt. Use right away or refrigerate for up to 1 day. Serve very cold.

PER SERVING	
Calories: 81	
Protein: 4 g	
Fat: 4 g	
Carbohydrate: 9 g	
Fiber: 2 g	
Excellent source: Vitamin C, Folic Acid	
Good source: Vitamin A, Iron	

Dilled Squash Soup

Ripe apples sweeten this easy soup naturally. Wonderful to have in the freezer to haul out for a spontaneous dinner party, or to enjoy in front of the TV with a thick slice of pumpernickel bread.

PREPARATION TIME: 35 MINUTES / MICROWAVING TIME: 4 MINUTES

COOKING TIME: 40 MINUTES / MAKES: 12 ONE-CUP SERVINGS

2 large acorn squashes, about 4 lbs (2 kg) in total

8 apples, peeled, cored and quartered, about 2½ lbs (1.25 kg)

2 large onions, chopped

4 cups chicken broth or bouillon, or vegetable broth

1 tbsp dried dill seed, or 2 tsp dried dillweed

½ tsp dried leaf thyme

½ tsp salt

2 cups milk, chicken broth or bouillon, or water

1. To make squash easier to peel, place 1 squash in the microwave and cook on high for 2 minutes. Repeat with remaining squash. Slice in half and remove seeds. Slice off peel and cut pulp into large cubes.

2. In a large saucepan, combine squash with remaining ingredients, except milk. Cover and bring to a boil over medium-high heat. Reduce heat and simmer, covered, stirring occasionally, until squash is very tender, about 35 minutes.

3. Using a blender or food processor, purée squash mixture in several batches. If serving right away, return purée to saucepan. Stir in milk, or additional bouillon or water until soup is the consistency you like. Cook, stirring often, over medium-low heat until hot, but not boiling.

ACORN SQUASH

INSTANT NOODLE SOUP BOOSTERS

Add to the goodness of popular instant noodle soups with these no-fuss stir-ins. Prepare soup according to package directions, then mix in:

- Bite-size pieces of leftover roast, cooked chicken or turkey, canned beans, cubes of tofu, small cooked shrimp, tuna or strips of deli meats for added protein.

- Shreds of Swiss chard, spinach or bok choy for extra nutrients.

- Microwaved, frozen mixed vegetables for added fiber.

- Finely chopped red pepper, or cooked sweet potato or carrot for a beta-carotene boost.

PER SERVING

Calories:	138
Protein:	4 g
Fat:	2 g
Carbohydrate:	29 g
Fiber:	5 g

MAKE AHEAD: *Pour squash purée into containers or resealable plastic bags. Do not add milk. Soup can be refrigerated for 2 days or frozen for months. To reheat, pour a little water in bottom of a saucepan just wide enough to hold frozen soup. Add soup. Cover and reheat slowly, stirring often. When piping hot, stir in milk, water or bouillon until soup is the consistency you like. Or, put 2 cups of frozen soup in a large bowl, cover and microwave on high for 8 to 10 minutes. Stir after 4 minutes, then every 2 minutes. When hot, stir in milk or additional broth or water until it's the consistency you like. Then, continue microwaving until hot.*

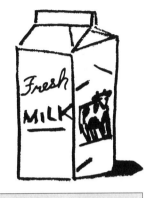

SOUP'S ON

Soul-satisfying soups can be made in minutes without using a dry-soup base. Just check out the speedy soups below. To make a warming supper, add slices of whole grain bread.

LIVELY ITALIAN LENTIL

Heat a 19-oz (540-mL) can Italian-style stewed tomatoes with a 10-oz (284-mL) can undiluted chicken broth or 1 cup chicken bouillon and 1½ cups water. Stir in ½ cup uncooked lentils. Cover and simmer, stirring often, until lentils are tender, about 35 minutes. *Makes 4½ cups.*

MEXICAN CUP OF SOUP

Stir 1 teaspoon salsa and 1 teaspoon light sour cream into 1 cup piping hot tomato soup. *Serves 1.*

SQUASH SIPPER

Heat a 12-oz (400-g) pkg frozen puréed squash with 2 cups chicken bouillon and ½ teaspoon dried dillweed or curry. When hot, but not boiling, stir in ¼ to ½ cup light sour cream or yogurt. *Makes 3¼ cups.*

LIGHT CHILI SOUP

Heat 1 cup spaghetti sauce with 1 cup water, 1 teaspoon chili powder, ¼ teaspoon garlic powder or 2 crushed garlic cloves, ¼ teaspoon hot red pepper flakes and a 19-oz (540-mL) can drained white or red kidney beans. Cover and simmer for 5 minutes, or until hot. *Makes 3½ cups.*

INSTANT BORSCHT

Drain liquid from a 10-oz (284-mL) can of beets into a saucepan. Add 1½ cups vegetable cocktail juice, and heat. Shred beets and add them to pan, along with 2 cups finely shredded cabbage. Cover and simmer, stirring once, until cabbage is tender, about 5 minutes. *Makes 3 cups.*

BROCCOLI BOOSTER

Purée 3 cups well-cooked broccoli with a 10-oz (284-mL) can chicken broth and ½ teaspoon curry powder or cumin. Heat, then stir in ¼ to ½ cup yogurt or light sour cream. Heat until hot, but do not boil. *Makes 2½ cups.*

Curried Harvest Pumpkin Soup

Fragrant with cumin and the fresh scent of apples, this thick satiny soup is perfect to begin a fall dinner or to serve as a simple meal.

PREPARATION TIME: 15 MINUTES / COOKING TIME: 30 MINUTES

MAKES: 6 ONE-CUP SERVINGS

EASY HOMEMADE STOCK

Break up turkey or chicken bones and put in a large saucepan. Add several sliced onions, sliced carrots, celery stalks with leaves, a few whole peppercorns and large pinches of salt, thyme, sage and savory. Cover with water. Cover and bring to a gentle boil. Continue boiling, stirring occasionally, for at least 3 hours. Strain broth and discard vegetables and bones. Keep stock refrigerated.

For easy storage, concentrate stock by boiling, uncovered, until reduced by half or two-thirds. Freeze in small quantities in freezer bags or in reusable containers.

4 sweet apples, such as McIntosh
1 tbsp butter or olive oil
1 onion, finely chopped
2 crushed garlic cloves
1 tbsp curry powder
1 tsp ground cumin
14-oz (398-mL) can pumpkin purée (not pie filling)
4 cups chicken broth or bouillon, or vegetable broth
1 cup water
1 tsp granulated sugar
Low-fat yogurt or light sour cream
Chopped fresh coriander

1. Peel and chop apples. You should have about 3 cups. Melt butter in a large saucepan set over medium heat. Add onion, garlic, curry powder and cumin. Sauté, stirring occasionally, until onion has softened and mixture is very fragrant, about 5 minutes. Stir in apples, pumpkin, broth, water and sugar. Bring to a boil, stirring often, then cover and reduce heat to low. Simmer, stirring occasionally, for 25 minutes.

2. Purée soup in a food processor or blender. Return to saucepan and reheat, covered, over low heat until hot. Whisk in yogurt or light sour cream to taste. Or serve with a swirl of yogurt in the center and a scattering of coriander sprigs. Covered and refrigerated, soup will keep well for up to 3 days and freezes well.

PER SERVING

Calories: 131

Protein: 5 g

Fat: 4 g

Carbohydrate: 22 g

Fiber: 4 g

Excellent source: Vitamin A

Rona's Roasted Tomato Soup

Chatelaine's editor Rona Maynard likes to roast tomatoes to give them a caramelized taste before whirling them into a soup. The result is rich tasting but low-fat. In the fall, make up a big batch for the freezer.

PREPARATION TIME: 15 MINUTES / ROASTING TIME: 35 MINUTES
MAKES: 6 HALF-CUP SERVINGS

2 lbs (1 kg) plum tomatoes
3 garlic cloves
1 to 2 tsp sugar
½ tsp salt
¼ tsp freshly ground black pepper
10-oz (284-mL) can chicken broth, undiluted, or 1 cup chicken bouillon or vegetable broth
1 tsp balsamic vinegar, or 2 tsp sherry
1 tsp dried basil, or ½ cup chopped fresh basil
Light sour cream (optional)

1. Move oven rack to highest level and preheat oven to 450°F (230°C). Cut tomatoes in half, lengthwise. Place tomatoes, skin-side down, in a single layer on ungreased cookie sheets. Scatter whole peeled garlic cloves around tomatoes. Sprinkle tomatoes with 1 teaspoon sugar, salt and pepper. Roast, uncovered, until tomato edges are brown tinged, about 35 minutes.

2. Purée roasted tomatoes and garlic in a food processor, adding chicken broth as needed to keep mixture from sticking. Whirl until almost smooth. Stir in any remaining chicken broth and vinegar. If using dried basil, stir in. Taste and add remaining teaspoon sugar, if needed.

3. Serve right away. Or, refrigerate for up to 3 days or freeze. If using fresh basil, stir in just before serving. Serve hot or cold with a swirl of sour cream.

PROTEIN-PLUS SOUP

In a frying pan, cook 1 chopped sweet pepper and 1 chopped onion with 2 slices chopped bacon over medium heat, stirring often, for 7 minutes. Add 10-oz (284-mL) can chicken broth, 19 oz (540 mL) tomatoes with juice, 19 oz (540 mL) Romano beans and 1 teaspoon dried leaf thyme. Simmer for 10 minutes. *Makes 5 cups.*

PER SERVING

Calories: 50
Protein: 4 g
Fat: 1 g
Carbohydrate: 8 g
Fiber: 2 g
Good source: Vitamin A, Vitamin C

Spring Chicken and Asparagus Soup

Asparagus, slivers of mushrooms and bits of red pepper in a soothing broth add up to a sophisticated and low-calorie spring starter.

ASPARAGUS: GUILT-FREE FINGER FOOD

The best asparagus is fresh asparagus. Look for bright green, straight, firm stalks with tightly closed, compact tips. Choose spears that are at least a quarter of an inch in diameter. Avoid those with large, woody, hard, white bases. This is one splurge — minus the hollandaise — that is guilt-free: eight cooked spears contain almost no fat, about 30 calories and a healthy supply of vitamin C, folic acid and fiber. Indulge!

PREPARATION TIME: 10 MINUTES / COOKING TIME: 8 MINUTES

MAKES: 7 ONE-CUP SERVINGS

2 (10-oz/284-mL) cans chicken broth, preferably lower-salt

¼ cup dry sherry

1 tbsp freshly squeezed lemon juice

¼ tsp salt

4 thin slices fresh ginger

¼ lb (125 g) mixed fresh mushrooms, such as shiitake, oyster or button

2 cups diagonally sliced asparagus (1-inch pieces)

1 small red pepper, seeded and finely chopped

2 green onions, thinly sliced

1 cup diced cooked chicken

1. Empty broth into a saucepan. Add 2 soup cans of water, sherry, lemon juice, salt and ginger. Bring to a boil over medium heat. Meanwhile, thinly slice mushrooms.

2. When broth is boiling gently, stir in all vegetables and chicken. Continue cooking, uncovered and stirring occasionally, until vegetables are done as you like, about 5 minutes. Remove ginger and serve.

PER SERVING

Calories:	71
Protein:	7 g
Fat:	2 g
Carbohydrate:	6 g
Fiber:	1 g
Excellent source:	Folic Acid
Good source:	Vitamin C

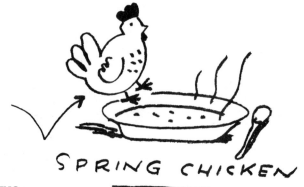

SPRING CHICKEN

Two-Tone Melon Soup

Here's an impressive answer when you want a light and pretty soup to start a summer party. Cantaloupe and honeydew purées get equal billing in a wide soup bowl with a designer's swirl of yogurt joining the two.

PREPARATION TIME: 10 MINUTES / REFRIGERATION TIME: 4 HOURS
MAKES: 4 ONE-CUP SERVINGS

½ large ripe cantaloupe
½ large ripe honeydew melon
4 tsp freshly squeezed lime juice
¼ cup yogurt or light sour cream (optional)
Fresh mint leaves (optional)

1. Scoop out melon seeds. Peel melons and cut into chunks. Put only cantaloupe pieces in a blender or food processor. Whirl until puréed. Pour into a bowl.

2. Purée honeydew and pour into a second bowl. Stir 1 to 2 teaspoons lime juice into each soup. Then, if you like, whisk 2 tablespoons yogurt into one or both soups. Or yogurt can be swirled in the soup when it's served. Refrigerate until well chilled, about 4 hours. They will keep well for at least 1 day.

3. To serve, pour each soup into a separate measuring cup. Then simultaneously pour each soup into opposite sides of the same wide soup dish. Do not mix. If you haven't whisked yogurt into the soups, swirl a little yogurt in the center of the bowl letting it run between the two soups. A mint garnish is nice.

MELON MANIA
Cantaloupe is one of the most nutritionally well-rounded fruits. One-half a melon, at about 90 calories, contains more than your daily requirement of vitamin C, is loaded with beta-carotene, folic acid and potassium and is virtually fat-free. A ripe cantaloupe should give slightly on its blossom end (opposite from stem end) when pushed, but should not be mushy. When choosing your melon, don't hesitate to sniff. It should have a sweet, musky aroma. If it isn't ripe, leave it on the counter until it ripens. It's overripe if seeds can be heard sloshing around when you shake it.

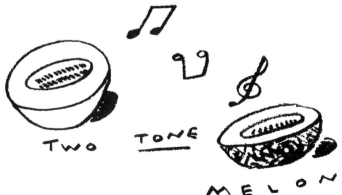

PER SERVING

Calories: 85	
Protein: 1 g	
Fat: Trace	
Carbohydrate: 22 g	
Fiber: 2 g	
Excellent source: Vitamin A, Vitamin C, Folic Acid	

Bloody Mary Soup with Vodka

TOMATO SMARTS

Buy:
Choose heavy, firm, slightly supple tomatoes.

Ripen:
Never ripen tomatoes on a windowsill — tomatoes will dry out. Seal them in a brown paper bag with an apple or pear, which produces a natural gas that speeds up ripening.

Store:
Keep at room temperature.

Freeze:
Cut stem ends from ripe unpeeled tomatoes, then freeze tomatoes. Frozen tomatoes can be held under hot running water and skins will slip off. Use in soups, stews and sauces.

Slice:
How you cut tomatoes makes a difference. Slicing from stem to bottom keeps more juice in the tomatoes.

This sophisticated garden-fresh soup is a perfect barbecue opener. Use the recipe as a guide. Adjust to taste as you would when whipping up a drink. If you can't find ripe tomatoes, use canned — they're always chock-full of flavor and nutrients. Serve with long skinny bread sticks.

PREPARATION TIME: 10 MINUTES
REFRIGERATION TIME: 30 MINUTES / MAKES: 6 HALF-CUP SERVINGS

4 large ripe tomatoes, peeled, seeded and coarsely chopped
1 cup tomato juice, tomato-clam juice, or vegetable cocktail juice
¼ cup finely chopped celery
1 tsp lemon juice
1 tsp granulated sugar
½ tsp Worcestershire sauce
¼ tsp garlic salt, or 1 small crushed garlic clove
Pinches of dried leaf thyme and basil
Dash of hot pepper sauce
1 to 2 tbsp vodka (optional)
Light sour cream and chopped fresh basil (optional)

1. Combine all ingredients, except sour cream and fresh basil, in a blender or food processor. Whirl until fairly smooth. Refrigerate until very cold. Soup will keep well for several days. Serve with a swirl of sour cream and a sprinkle of fresh basil.

PER SERVING

Calories: 32	
Protein: 1 g	
Fat: Trace	
Carbohydrate: 6 g	
Fiber: 1 g	
Good source: Vitamin C	

Roasted Red Pepper Soup

The unique, smoky, slightly sweet flavor of roasted peppers is the essence of this healthy puréed soup. A knock-'em-dead beginning for any festive dinner.

PREPARATION TIME: 20 MINUTES / BAKING TIME: 36 MINUTES

COOKING TIME: 16 MINUTES / MAKES: 8 HALF-CUP SERVINGS

4 large red peppers
1 to 2 tbsp good-quality olive oil
2 crushed garlic cloves
2 onions, chopped
3 cups chicken broth or bouillon
Freshly ground black pepper

1. Preheat oven to 375°F (190°C). Place whole peppers on a baking sheet and roast for 18 minutes. Turn peppers and continue roasting for 18 more minutes. Remove peppers from baking sheet and place them in a paper bag. Seal it and let it stand until peppers are cool enough to handle, about 10 minutes. Remove peppers from bag and peel off skins. Slice peppers in half and remove seeds. Cut into large chunks and set aside. Refrigerate if making ahead.

2. In a large saucepan, heat oil over medium heat. Add garlic and onions, and sauté until onions are very soft, about 8 minutes. Stir in roasted peppers and continue cooking until peppers are very soft. Put cooked pepper mixture in a food processor fitted with a metal blade. Whirl, using an on-and-off motion, until blended and smooth. Return puréed mixture to saucepan and add chicken broth. Cover and cook over medium heat, stirring occasionally, for about 8 to 10 minutes, until soup is warm. Sprinkle with black pepper. Spoon into soup bowls and garnish with a swirl of sour cream in the center. Soup will keep well for at least 2 days in refrigerator and also freezes well.

SPICY LENTIL SOUP

Rinse 1 cup canned lentils and place in a large saucepan with 1 coarsely chopped onion, 3 crushed garlic cloves, 2 teaspoons curry powder, $\frac{1}{8}$ teaspoon crushed hot red pepper flakes, 2 (10-oz/284-mL) cans undiluted chicken broth and 2 cups water. Cover and bring to boil over high heat. Reduce heat and boil gently until lentils are soft, 5 to 10 minutes. Swirl a large dollop of yogurt in each bowl. *Makes 4 cups.*

PER SERVING

Calories: 57	
Protein: 3 g	
Fat: 2 g	
Carbohydrate: 7 g	
Fiber: 2 g	
Excellent source: Vitamin C	
Good source: Vitamin A	

Getaway Caribbean Chowder

Here's an express way to make your own fish stock and chowder. A big colorful bowl of this seductive soup laced with mango, red pepper and tender red snapper reels in only 192 calories.

PREPARATION TIME: 15 MINUTES / COOKING TIME: 35 MINUTES

MAKES: 5 TWO-CUP SERVINGS

PER SERVING

Calories: 192

Protein: 25 g

Fat: 4 g

Carbohydrate: 15 g

Fiber: 2 g

Excellent source: Vitamin A, Vitamin C

FAST STOCK

1 each of celery stalk with leaves, carrot, onion and bay leaf

1½- to 2-lb (750-g to 1-kg) whole red snapper, filleted and skinned, with bones and head reserved

8 cups water

MORE CHEERY CHOWDERS

SPICY CORN AND SHRIMP CHOWDER

In a 10-cup (2.5-L) microwave-safe dish, put 1 finely chopped small onion, 1 finely chopped celery stalk, 1½ cups frozen kernel corn and 1 tablespoon olive oil. Microwave, covered, on high 4 minutes. Finely dice 2 potatoes and stir in along with 3 cups milk, ¼ teaspoon salt and generous pinches of black pepper, nutmeg and crushed hot red pepper flakes. Microwave, covered, until potatoes are tender, about 16 minutes. Stir once. Purée two-thirds of mixture, then pour into chowder in dish. Microwave, covered, until bubbling, about 7 minutes, stirring in ½ lb (250 g) peeled and deveined shrimp; add frozen shrimp for the last 5 minutes of cooking or fresh shrimp for the last 2 minutes. *Makes 5 cups.*

ITALIAN COUNTRY BEAN CHOWDER

Pour contents of 19-oz (540-mL) can Italian-style stewed tomatoes into a large saucepan placed over high heat. Add 19-oz (540-mL) can drained and rinsed kidney or Romano beans or chick-peas, 1 cup water and ½ teaspoon Italian seasoning or ½ teaspoon each of dried basil or leaf oregano. Coarsely chop 2 small zucchini and add. When mixture boils, add ¾ lb (375 g) fresh fish fillets or a 1-lb (400-g) package frozen fillets (rinsed under cold water and drained). Reduce heat to medium and cook, covered and stirring often, until fish is hot and flakes easily with a fork, about 3 minutes for fresh, up to 10 minutes for frozen fish. Break fish into bite-size pieces. *Makes 7 cups.*

SOUP

1 onion, chopped

1 crushed garlic clove

1 sweet red or green pepper

1 jalapeño pepper or small pieces of Scotch
bonnet pepper, seeded

2 ripe tomatoes

1 ripe mango

2 tbsp freshly squeezed lime juice, about 1 lime

1 tsp salt

¼ tsp freshly ground black pepper

Fresh coriander or parsley leaves

1. To make stock, cut celery, carrot and 1 onion into large chunks. Put in a large pot with bay leaf, fish bones and head, and water. Bring to a boil over high heat. Skim off any foam. Reduce heat to low and simmer, uncovered, without stirring, for 20 minutes. Strain. Save fish stock and discard vegetables and bones. You should have about 7 cups of stock.

2. To make chowder, return 1 cup stock to pot along with 1 chopped onion and garlic. Set over medium heat. Seed and chop sweet pepper. Finely chop jalapeño pepper. Add to soup. Simmer until onion has softened, about 7 minutes. Add remaining stock and bring to a boil over high heat.

3. Meanwhile, remove any bones from fish fillets and cut into bite-size chunks. Cut tomatoes in half. Squeeze out seeds and discard them. Dice tomatoes into ¼-inch pieces. Slice peel from mango, then cut pulp from stone. Chop pulp. Add fish to boiling soup. Reduce heat to medium and stir in tomatoes, mango, lime juice, salt and pepper. Heat until fish flakes easily with a fork and soup is hot, about 3 to 4 minutes. Scatter with fresh coriander or parsley leaves and serve.

**HOT PEPPERS:
HANDLE WITH CARE!**

Hot peppers are commonly used to give hot spicy food its kick. Capsaicin, the substance that makes hot peppers hot, also can cause a burning, stinging sensation on hands and eyes if you're not careful. Always wear rubber gloves when handling hot peppers. Rinse your cutting board and knife before removing the gloves. If you do get juice on your skin, a little milk on the affected area will provide relief. As a general rule, the smaller the pepper the hotter it is. The heat is concentrated in the veins or ribs near the seed heart, not in the seeds themselves. The seeds, however, do absorb the hotness from the veins.

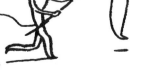

Quick Curried Lentil and Carrot Soup

Lentils are rich in protein and fiber and are nearly fat-free. A bowl of this soup has only 1 gram of fat and 110 calories and is an excellent source of vitamin A.

PREPARATION TIME: 10 MINUTES / COOKING TIME: 25 MINUTES

MAKES: 7 ONE-CUP SERVINGS

1 large onion

3 crushed garlic cloves

1 tsp curry powder

¼ tsp salt

3 cups chicken broth or bouillon, or vegetable broth

19-oz (540-mL) can lentils, or 1 cup uncooked lentils

3 to 4 carrots

2 celery stalks

2 large fresh tomatoes, or 4 canned tomatoes (optional)

½ cup light sour cream (optional)

1. Coarsely chop onion. Put onion in a large saucepan with garlic, curry powder and salt. Add broth and set pan over medium-high heat. Drain canned lentils or rinse dry lentils under cold running water and add them to onion mixture. Bring mixture to a boil, uncovered and stirring often.

2. Meanwhile, thinly slice carrots and celery and add to saucepan. When soup boils, reduce heat to low and simmer, covered, stirring occasionally, until vegetables and lentils are done as you like, about 20 minutes for canned lentils or 30 minutes for dry lentils.

3. Meanwhile, peel tomatoes, if you wish, and coarsely chop them. When vegetables are tender, stir tomatoes into soup and continue cooking until hot, about 5 minutes. When serving, swirl a dollop of sour cream into each bowl of soup. Serve with whole wheat bread.

FIBER FIXES

If you're getting your fiber fix from granola and mega-muffins, you may be getting more than you bargained for. A large, cakey muffin may contain 6 to 8 g of fiber (about one-quarter of your daily requirement), but it can also contain 350 to 500 calories, with most of the calories coming from fat. Half a cup of granola has about 300 calories and usually 50% of the calories come from fat. You can get the same amount of fiber without all the fat (and calories) from a bowl of bran cereal and low-fat milk. The best way to include more dietary fiber is by eating more fresh fruits and vegetables and whole grains — foods such as pears, raspberries, carrots, oats and lentils.

PER SERVING

Calories: 110

Protein: 8 g

Fat: 1 g

Carbohydrate: 18 g

Fiber: 4 g

Excellent source: Vitamin A, Folic Acid

Good source: Iron

Smart Salads

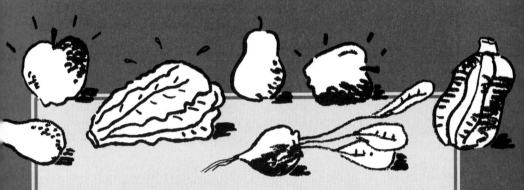

Zesty Two-Tone Potato Salad

Moroccan Spicy Carrot and Mint Salad

Garden Veggie Lentil Salad

Sophisticated Beet and Celeriac Salad

Healthy Greek Luncheon Salad

Oriental Pasta Salad

Fresh Mint, Tomato and Coriander Tabbouleh Salad

Sweet 'n' Sour Coleslaw

Lynne's Garden Tomato Salad

Zesty Two-Tone Potato Salad

Potato salads are a perennial barbecue favorite. We like to serve this deliciously healthy mix of beta-carotene–rich sweet potatoes, oranges and white potatoes as a barbecue sidekick.

PREPARATION TIME: 25 MINUTES / COOKING TIME: 20 MINUTES

MAKES: 10 CUPS

2 to 3 large sweet potatoes, about 2 lbs (1 kg)
4 thin-skinned white potatoes, about 2 lbs (1 kg)
2 to 3 oranges
¼ cup olive oil
2 tbsp freshly squeezed lemon juice
1 tbsp Dijon mustard
1 tbsp granulated sugar
2 crushed garlic cloves
½ tsp salt
¼ tsp freshly ground black pepper
Chives, coriander or parsley (optional)

1. To prepare potatoes, cut sweet potatoes in half and leave white potatoes whole. Put sweet potatoes in one saucepan and white potatoes in another. Cover potatoes with water and bring to a boil over medium-high heat. Boil gently, partially covered, until potatoes are just tender when pierced with a skewer, about 20 to 30 minutes. To keep sweet potatoes from becoming mushy, remove them from water while they are still fairly firm, since they continue to cook after being removed from heat.

2. Or to microwave potatoes, slice sweet potatoes into quarters, lengthwise. Place cut-side down on paper towels, with thickest parts to outside. Microwave on high until barely tender when pierced with a fork, about 9 minutes. Do not overcook or potatoes will be mushy. Microwave whole white potatoes just until tender, about 12 minutes.

ELEGANT MIXED GREENS WITH CHAMPAGNE VINAIGRETTE

Marjorie Agnew, owner of The Main Course cookware shop in North York, Ont., dresses up her big-scale party salads with a classy champagne dressing. She whisks 1 tablespoon of Dijon mustard with 2 tablespoons of white-wine vinegar or champagne vinegar, then slowly whisks in ¼ cup cold champagne followed by ½ to ¾ cup olive oil, and salt and pepper to taste. She tosses this with mixed salad greens, radicchio and toasted pine nuts. *Makes about 1 cup dressing for a salad for 12.*

PER CUP

Calories:	196
Protein:	3 g
Fat:	6 g
Carbohydrate:	35 g
Fiber:	3 g
Excellent source:	Vitamin A, Vitamin C

3. Meanwhile, finely grate peel from 1 orange. Squeeze 1 cup juice from oranges and pour it into a large bowl. Whisk in peel, oil, lemon juice, Dijon, sugar, garlic, salt and pepper. Peel the warm potatoes and cut into 1½-inch pieces, adding warm pieces to dressing as they are cut. When all potatoes have been added, stir gently. Sprinkle snipped chives or chopped coriander or parsley over salad just before serving. Salad can be served right away, but flavor will be better if refrigerated for at least a few hours or overnight. Covered and refrigerated, salad will keep well for at least 3 days. Serve at room temperature.

Moroccan Spicy Carrot and Mint Salad

Moroccan meals, even breakfast, feature a selection of interesting cold vegetable dishes like this carrot salad, lightly coated with a honey-lemon dressing. You'll be surprised at how such ordinary inexpensive ingredients create an extraordinary taste sensation.

PREPARATION TIME: 15 MINUTES / COOKING TIME: 10 MINUTES
MAKES: 4½ CUPS

5 to 6 carrots

1 onion

3 tbsp olive oil

1½ tsp ground cumin

¼ tsp each of paprika, salt and freshly ground black pepper

Pinch of cayenne pepper

2 tbsp freshly squeezed lemon juice

2 tsp liquid honey

2 tbsp chopped fresh mint or 1 to 2 tsp dried crushed mint leaves

SENSATIONAL SPINACH AND PEAR SALAD

Wash 1 large bunch or 10-oz (284-g) bag fresh spinach and dry. Remove stems. Tear leaves into bite-size pieces and place in a salad bowl. Core 1 firm but ripe pear or 2 small sugar pears. Thinly slice pear and add to spinach. Put 2 tablespoons chutney, preferably mango, in a small dish. If chutney contains any large chunks, remove them, finely chop and return to bowl. Stir in ¼ cup light Italian dressing. Just before serving, pour dressing over spinach and pears and toss until evenly coated. *Makes 4 servings.*

PER HALF CUP

Calories: 74	
Protein: 1 g	
Fat: 5 g	
Carbohydrate: 8 g	
Fiber: 2 g	
Excellent source: Vitamin A	

1. Peel carrots and slice them diagonally into ⅛-inch slices. You should have about 4 cups. Thinly slice onion. Heat 1 tablespoon oil in a large frying pan set over medium heat. When oil is hot, add onion and sprinkle with cumin, paprika, salt, pepper and cayenne. Sauté, stirring often, until onion is just softened and spices are very fragrant, about 3 minutes.

2. Add carrots and continue sautéing. Stir often until carrots are hot and just beginning to soften, about 7 minutes. Remove from heat and let them stand while continuing with recipe. The carrots will continue to cook from the heat of the pan.

3. In a large bowl, whisk lemon juice with honey until dissolved. Whisk in remaining 2 tablespoons oil. Add hot carrot mixture and toss until coated. Cool to room temperature. Toss with mint and serve salad at room temperature. Refrigerated it will keep for 3 days. Great with chicken and mashed potatoes.

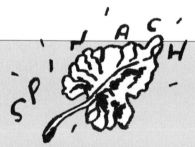

SMALL PERFECT SALADS

CURRIED PEA SALAD

Cook a 10-oz (300-g) package frozen peas according to package directions. Drain and rinse under cold running water until cool. Stir ¼ cup low-fat mayonnaise with 1 teaspoon curry powder. Stir into peas. Taste and add more curry if needed. Refrigerate until chilled or up to 1 day. Stir in 2 cups shredded fresh spinach leaves before serving. Season with salt and pepper. *Serves 4.*

TUNA-NECTARINE TOSS

Break 1 head Bibb lettuce into bite-size pieces and place in a large salad bowl. Drain 2 (6½-oz/184-g) cans tuna. Chop 2 nectarines or peaches and slice 2 stalks celery. Sprinkle them over lettuce. Stir ¾ cup low-fat sour cream or mayonnaise with ¾ teaspoon curry powder and 2 tablespoons chutney. Taste and add more curry, salt and pepper if needed. Pour over salad and toss. *Serves 4.*

WARM SPINACH AND CHÈVRE SALAD FOR TWO

Cut 2 slices of bacon into ½-inch pieces. Place them on a microwave-safe plate, not paper towels. Microwave on high until crisp, about 2 minutes. Meanwhile, tear 3 cups of fresh spinach leaves into bite-size pieces. Place in a bowl. Crumble ¼ cup of creamy chèvre over top. When bacon is cooked, pour 1 teaspoon of bacon fat into a small bowl. Whisk in 2 teaspoons olive oil, 1 teaspoon balsamic vinegar and pinches of salt and pepper. Microwave, uncovered, on high for 30 seconds until hot. Drizzle over salad and toss until coated. Sprinkle with bacon. *Serves 2.*

Garden Veggie Lentil Salad

Lentils cook "from scratch" in 30 minutes. This salad has an exceptionally good texture, lively earthy flavor and enough protein to serve as dinner.

PREPARATION TIME: 10 MINUTES / COOKING TIME: 30 MINUTES

MAKES: 3 CUPS

1 cup dried green or brown lentils

1 large onion, preferably red

2 tbsp olive oil

3 crushed garlic cloves

2 peppers, 1 red and 1 green, seeded and chopped

2 carrots, peeled and chopped

2 tbsp balsamic or cider vinegar

1½ tsp ground cumin or curry powder

½ tsp salt

¼ tsp cayenne pepper (optional)

½ cup chopped fresh coriander (optional)

1. Rinse lentils under cold running water. Place them in a saucepan and cover with water, about 1 inch above lentils. Cover and quickly bring to a boil over high heat. Reduce heat to low and simmer until lentils are tender but not mushy, about 30 minutes. Add more boiling water, if necessary, to keep lentils covered during cooking time.

2. Meanwhile, finely chop onion. Heat 1 tablespoon oil in a large frying pan set over medium heat. Add onion and garlic. Sauté, stirring occasionally, until onion is softened, about 5 minutes. Stir in chopped peppers and carrots and sauté for 2 minutes. Remove from heat and turn into a salad bowl.

3. When lentils are tender, drain well and add to vegetable mixture. Whisk 1 tablespoon oil with vinegar and seasonings. Stir into salad until lentils are evenly coated. Sprinkle with chopped fresh coriander, if you like. Salad can be made completely ahead of time and refrigerated for up to 2 days.

CURRIED LENTIL SALAD

Drain a 19-oz (540-mL) can of lentils, then rinse with cold water. In a bowl, stir ½ cup light sour cream with ½ teaspoon curry powder and ½ teaspoon salt. Stir in lentils, then about 2 cups of chopped vegetables, such as finely chopped carrot, sweet peppers, thinly sliced celery, green onions and chopped coriander. You can serve right away, but the flavor is better if refrigerated overnight. *Serves 4.*

PER HALF CUP

Calories: 162

Protein: 9 g

Fat: 5 g

Carbohydrate: 22 g

Fiber: 5 g

Excellent source: Folic Acid, Iron

Sophisticated Beet and Celeriac Salad

This beautiful ruby-colored salad of julienned vegetables could serve as the centerpiece of any entertaining fall dinner, especially Thanksgiving. Make it a day ahead if you like. It won't wilt and the flavor may even intensify.

PREPARATION TIME: 45 MINUTES / COOKING TIME: 40 MINUTES

MAKES: 12 CUPS

6 beets

6 carrots

2 small celeriac (celery root)

⅓ cup olive oil

3 tbsp cider vinegar

1 tbsp Dijon mustard

1 tbsp liquid honey

2 tsp curry powder

½ tsp salt

¼ tsp freshly ground black pepper

½ cup chopped fresh coriander (optional)

1. Trim leaves from beets but do not skin them. Place whole beets in a saucepan and cover with water. Cover saucepan and bring water to a boil over high heat. Reduce heat to medium-low and boil gently, covered, until beets are tender when pierced with a fork or skewer, about 30 to 40 minutes.

2. Meanwhile, peel carrots. Slice into very thin strips, about 1½ inches long. Peel celeriac and slice it into similar-size strips. Bring a large pot of water to a full rolling boil over high heat. Add carrot and celeriac strips. As soon as water returns to a full boil, after about 2 to 3 minutes, drain vegetables and immediately rinse them with cold running water to stop the cooking. Set aside to drain.

HIGH-PROTEIN LUNCHBOX SALAD

In a container with a tight-fitting lid or in a resealable plastic bag, combine 1 cup rinsed canned or cooked beans (such as kidney, Romano or chick-peas) with ¼ cup mild salsa, ¼ teaspoon cumin, 1 thinly sliced celery stalk and 1 thinly sliced green onion. Gently stir together. Refrigerate salad, if making it the night before. It will keep well for several days or at room temperature for at least 1 day. Pack slices of vegetables, such as carrots, peppers and cucumber, to munch with the salad, a wholewheat roll and a big pear or apple for dessert.

PER HALF CUP

Calories:	46
Protein:	1 g
Fat:	3 g
Carbohydrate:	5 g
Fiber:	1 g
Excellent Source:	Vitamin A

3. Measure oil, vinegar, Dijon, honey, curry powder, salt and pepper into a large bowl. Whisk ingredients until blended. When beets are tender, drain and rinse with cold water. Rub beets with your fingers to remove skins. Slice beets into very thin strips.

4. Add beets, carrots and celeriac to dressing. Sprinkle salad with coriander. Stir gently to mix and to evenly coat vegetables with dressing. For best taste, serve at room temperature. Covered and refrigerated, salad will keep well for up to 2 days.

Healthy Greek Luncheon Salad

We designed this wilt-proof rice salad as a lower-fat lunchtime treat you can carry in a brown bag or briefcase, and it beats anything from the fast-food counter for taste and price.

PREPARATION TIME: 5 MINUTES / MAKES: 1 SERVING

1 cup cooked rice
1 tbsp light Italian dressing
1 tomato, seeded and chopped
1 green onion, thinly sliced
¼ cup crumbled feta or creamy chèvre
½ cup cucumber chunks (optional)
Dried leaf oregano and garlic powder

1. Place rice in a container with a tight-fitting lid or in a resealable plastic bag. Stir in dressing. Add tomato along with green onion, cheese and cucumber, if using. Sprinkle salad with about ¼ teaspoon oregano and a generous pinch of garlic powder. Mix well. Taste and, if needed, stir in 1 more tablespoon dressing or about 1 teaspoon lemon juice. Seal tightly and salad is ready to go into a bag or your briefcase. To complete lunch, tuck in a whole wheat pita and piece of fruit. If making salad the night before, refrigerate it. Salad will keep well at room temperature for at least 4 hours.

PER SERVING

Calories: 384	
Protein: 11 g	
Fat: 8 g	
Carbohydrate: 66 g	
Fiber: 3 g	
Good source: Vitamin C, Folic Acid, Calcium	

Oriental Pasta Salad

Chock-full of colorful vegetables with a surprise of exotic mango, this beautiful pasta salad rings in at about 3 grams of fat per cup.

PREPARATION TIME: 30 MINUTES / COOKING TIME: 10 MINUTES
REFRIGERATION TIME: 3 HOURS / MAKES: 10 CUPS

½ (1-lb/450-g) pkg spaghetti or spaghettini, a bunch about 1 inch in diameter

2 red or yellow peppers, or 1 of each

1 large English cucumber

1 large mango, ripe but firm

1 tbsp each of olive oil and sesame oil, preferably dark

2 tbsp soy sauce

2 tbsp rice vinegar or white-wine vinegar

1 tbsp brown sugar

1 tbsp finely chopped fresh ginger

½ tsp salt

Pinch of cayenne pepper

2 green onions, thinly sliced

¼ cup chopped fresh coriander

PER CUP

Calories: 146

Protein: 4 g

Fat: 3 g

Carbohydrate: 26 g

Fiber: 2 g

Excellent Source: Vitamin C

Good Source: Vitamin A

HEALTHY SALAD DRESSINGS

Drizzling a basic vinaigrette over a few greens can add a lot of fat-laden calories and little else to a seemingly innocent side salad. But there are lots of ways to use nutritious ingredients to make a healthy dressing, starting, for example, with calcium-rich low-fat buttermilk or protein-rich cheese. Low-fat sour cream or light yogurt can also be used as a creamy base for dressing.

BUTTERMILK-TARRAGON

Stir ¼ cup buttermilk and ¼ cup low-fat sour cream with ¼ teaspoon dried tarragon or 1 teaspoon chopped fresh tarragon. *Makes ½ cup.*

FAST HERBED CHÈVRE

Mash 3 tablespoons creamy chèvre with 3 tablespoons yogurt. Stir in 1 tablespoon chopped fresh basil or ¼ teaspoon dried basil and a grinding of black pepper. *Makes ⅓ cup.*

GARLIC BALSAMIC

Stir 1 tablespoon balsamic or red-wine vinegar with ½ teaspoon Dijon mustard, 1 crushed garlic clove and generous pinches of hot red pepper flakes, basil and oregano. Gradually whisk in 3 tablespoons olive oil. Drizzle over romaine lettuce. *Makes ¼ cup.*

1. Bring a large pot of salted water to a full rolling boil over high heat. Add pasta, stirring to separate. Boil, uncovered and stirring occasionally, until al dente, about 11 minutes for spaghetti and 8 minutes for spaghettini. Do not overcook. Pour spaghetti into a strainer and rinse under cold running water until cool. Drain well and place in a large bowl.

2. Meanwhile, seed and thinly slice peppers. Cut cucumber in half, lengthwise, and thinly slice. Peel mango and slice fruit away from stone in pieces as large as possible. Then cut into bite-size strips.

3. To prepare dressing, whisk oils with soy sauce, vinegar, brown sugar, ginger, salt and cayenne. Pour dressing over pasta as soon as it has drained and toss until evenly coated. Add vegetables and mango if serving within 3 hours. Gently stir until evenly mixed. Salad can be served right away but flavor improves if refrigerated for at least 3 or 4 hours, or overnight. Salad looks wonderful served in the center of a bed of greens, sprinkled with sliced green onions and chopped fresh coriander.

MAKE AHEAD: *If you're refrigerating salad overnight, you may wish to add mango and cucumber just before or up to a few hours before serving to maintain their textures.*

MAKE FAT COUNT

When using fat in a recipe, consider using one with flavor. Using a richly flavored oil such as olive oil in a salad dressing, instead of a flavorless vegetable oil, not only provides a silky coating for the salad greens but gives a seductive flavor to each bite. When oiling vegetables or chicken for the barbecue, use olive oil or a mix of olive oil and a little sesame oil.

SASSY COLESLAW

Stir together ½ cup plain yogurt, 1 tablespoon white-wine vinegar, ½ teaspoon celery seed, ½ tsp regular mustard and a generous pinch of sugar. Toss with shredded cabbage. *Makes ½ cup.*

LIGHT BLUE CHEESE

Mash 2 tablespoons blue or Gorgonzola cheese with ⅓ cup low-fat sour cream, 1 tablespoon lemon juice and a generous pinch of black pepper. Great with greens and chopped chives. *Makes ½ cup.*

POTATO SALAD

Stir ½ cup light sour cream with 1 tablespoon grated onion, 1 tablespoon cider vinegar and ¼ teaspoon pepper. Toss with warm potatoes. *Makes ½ cup.*

EASY DIJON

Mash 2 tablespoons feta with 1 teaspoon Dijon mustard and 1 tablespoon balsamic vinegar. Gradually whisk in ¼ cup olive oil and a pinch of sugar. *Makes ⅓ cup.*

Fresh Mint, Tomato and Coriander Tabbouleh Salad

Our version of this refreshing Middle Eastern salad, unlike so many you buy, is tangy with lemon and full of the fresh taste of mint and garden tomatoes — making it perfect hot-weather picnic fare. Stir it together in the morning so the fresh herb flavors have a chance to thoroughly spread throughout the healthy bulgur. And this is a great potluck salad choice since it doesn't contain mayonnaise, so it travels well and doesn't have to be icy cold to be good.

PREPARATION TIME: 20 MINUTES / SOAKING TIME: 30 MINUTES

MAKES: 8 CUPS

1¾ cups medium or coarse bulgur, about
    8 oz (250 g)
3 cups boiling water
2 tbsp olive oil
½ cup freshly squeezed lemon juice, about
    2 large lemons
1 tsp salt
¼ tsp freshly ground black pepper
¼ tsp cayenne pepper (optional)
8 green onions, thinly sliced
½ cup coarsely chopped fresh coriander
    or parsley
½ cup chopped fresh mint
4 firm but ripe tomatoes
2 banana peppers (optional)

1. Place bulgur in a medium-size heat-proof bowl and pour boiling water over it. Let stand at room temperature, uncovered, without stirring, until all water is absorbed and bulgur is just tender, about 30 to 45 minutes.

BULGUR

Bulgur, which is sold in most supermarkets, often in the rice section, is made from wheat berries that are steamed, then dried and cracked. Coarse bulgur is best for salads such as tabbouleh. Do not confuse bulgur with cracked wheat, which is made from the dried wheat berry that is cracked without steaming. Cracked wheat is generally used for porridge.

PARTY PANACHE

For a classy buffet, serve the tabbouleh salad (at right) in hollowed-out tomatoes. As an appetizer, serve it in hollowed-out cherry tomatoes or endive leaves.

PER CUP

Calories: 157

Protein: 5 g

Fat: 4 g

Carbohydrate: 29 g

Fiber: 7 g

Good source: Vitamin C, Folic Acid

2. Meanwhile, in a large bowl, whisk oil with lemon juice, salt, black pepper and cayenne, if using. When all bulgur is tender and water is absorbed, stir into dressing with green onions, coriander and mint. Stir until bulgur is evenly coated with dressing. Slice tomatoes in half and squeeze out all juice and seeds. Coarsely chop and add to bulgur. Seed peppers, if using. Finely chop and stir into salad. Taste, then add more salt, cayenne, mint or oil if needed. Refrigerate, covered, if not serving right away or for up to 1 day.

Sweet 'n' Sour Coleslaw

This classic sweet-and-sour coleslaw will feed a crowd. Make it ahead, because, like a good chili, it tastes even better the next day.

PREPARATION TIME: 20 MINUTES / COOKING TIME: 5 MINUTES
REFRIGERATION TIME: 4 HOURS / MAKES: 15 CUPS

DRESSING
¾ cup white vinegar
½ cup granulated sugar
¼ cup olive oil
1 tsp salt
1 tsp dry mustard
½ tsp celery seeds
½ small onion, grated

SALAD
1 large green cabbage
2 medium carrots
2 peppers, 1 red and 1 green (optional)
Finely chopped parsley or coriander

1. Measure all dressing ingredients into a medium-size saucepan. Set over medium-high heat and bring to a boil. Stir often to ensure that sugar is dissolved. As soon as mixture comes to a boil, pour it into a heat-proof container, preferably metal to speed up cooling, and refrigerate until cold, about 30 to 45 minutes.

CHOPPED MINT
Since mint darkens quickly once it's chopped, hold off putting into recipes until at least 3 or 4 hours before serving.

TABBOULEH TWIST
Bring 1 cup chicken bouillon to a boil. Stir in 1 to 2 teaspoons butter, ¼ teaspoon salt and 1 cup couscous. Cover and let stand for 5 minutes. Fluff with a fork. Stir in 3 diced tomatoes, 1 cup chopped cucumber, 3 thinly sliced green onions and ¼ cup finely chopped fresh basil or mint. Serve at room temperature with barbecued chicken. *Serves 4 to 6.*

PER CUP

Calories: 83	
Protein: 1 g	
Fat: 4 g	
Carbohydrate: 13 g	
Fiber: 2 g	
Excellent Source: Vitamin A, Vitamin C	
Good Source: Folic Acid	

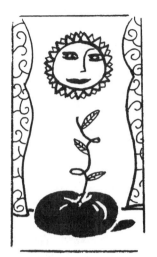

2. Meanwhile, using a large knife or the slicing disk of a food processor, thinly shred cabbage. Put it in a large bowl. You should have about 16 cups. Peel and grate carrots. Seed and thinly slice peppers, if using. Add carrots and peppers to cabbage, tossing until evenly mixed. Pour cooled dressing over vegetables and toss until coated.

3. Cover salad and refrigerate at least until chilled, about 4 hours or preferably overnight, to give flavors a chance to blend. Sprinkle with chopped parsley just before serving. Covered and refrigerated, this salad will keep for 3 or 4 days. Stir salad occasionally while it's in the refrigerator.

SUMMER SALAD DAYS

Warm weather spurs us on to load the fridge with salads that fit into any menu — brown-bag lunch, picnic or quick dinner. Crisp and crunchy, smooth and creamy, wet and spicy, these garden varieties are guaranteed to please.

THAI CUCUMBER

Thinly slice ½ unpeeled English cucumber. Mix 2 tablespoons boiling water with 2 tablespoons sugar until dissolved. Stir in 2 tablespoons white vinegar, ½ teaspoon hot chili paste and ¼ teaspoon salt. Pour over cucumbers. Keep refrigerated. *Makes 1½ cups.*

FRESH HERBED TABBOULEH

Cover 1 cup bulgur with boiling water. Let soak for 10 minutes. Drain well. Stir 1 tablespoon olive oil with 3 to 4 tablespoons lemon juice, 1 teaspoon each of sugar and salt, and a dash of hot pepper sauce if you wish. Stir into bulgur with 3 seeded and chopped tomatoes and ¼ cup each of chopped fresh parsley, mint, and chives or green onions. Serve right away or refrigerate, covered, for up to 2 days. *Makes 4 cups.*

CHERRY TOMATO

Slice 1 pint (500 mL) cherry tomatoes in half, crosswise. Mix with a 6-oz (170-mL) bottle of marinated artichokes, including dressing. Stir in pinches of salt, sugar and freshly ground black pepper. Serve over a bed of greens. Sprinkle with chopped parsley or chives. *Makes 4 cups.*

CURRIED CHICKEN

Stir ¼ cup light mayonnaise or sour cream with 1 tablespoon chutney and ¼ teaspoon curry powder. Mix 1 cup diced cooked chicken with ½ finely chopped apple or pear, 1 sliced green onion and 1 chopped celery stalk. Toss with dressing. Serve on a bed of salad greens. Keep refrigerated. *Makes 2¼ cups.*

GINGER PEACHY

Stir ½ cup plain yogurt with 1 teaspoon honey and a pinch of ground ginger. Stir in 2 sliced unpeeled peaches or nectarines. Serve right away or refrigerate, covered, for up to half a day. *Makes 2 cups.*

Lynne's Garden Tomato Salad

When a bumper crop's worth of garden-ripe tomatoes has you looking for new ways to serve them, try this simple salad full of fresh complex flavors. It's one you'll hanker for come January. This is the smart creation of Lynne Munkley, a CBC editor and a gardener par excellence.

PREPARATION TIME: 15 MINUTES / MAKES: 6 TO 8 SERVINGS

2 tbsp balsamic or red-wine vinegar

1 to 2 tbsp olive oil

1 large crushed garlic clove

¼ tsp each of salt and freshly ground black pepper

6 to 8 ripe tomatoes

1 small red onion

1 jalapeño pepper

¼ cup finely shredded or chopped fresh basil leaves

¼ to ½ cup crumbled chèvre (optional)

1. In a large mixing bowl, whisk vinegar with 1 tablespoon oil, garlic, salt and pepper.

2. Stir vegetables into dressing as they are cut. Slice tomatoes in half. Holding each one over the sink, squeeze out all its seeds and juice. Core and cut them into 1-inch chunks. Very thinly slice onion and separate it into rings. Finely chop jalapeño pepper. When all the vegetables have been added to the dressing, use a large spoon to gently toss. Taste and add more oil and a little sugar if needed. (If made ahead, salad can be left at room temperature for about an hour. After that, it will start to become watery.)

3. When ready to serve, gently stir in basil then sprinkle with chèvre, if you wish. Wonderful served on a bed of mixed greens with a crusty bread to sop up the juices.

TOMATO, SHALLOT AND BASIL SALAD

Sprinkle 3 thinly sliced ripe tomatoes with freshly ground black pepper, 2 tablespoons finely chopped shallots, 1 to 2 tablespoons olive oil, a spritz of balsamic or red-wine vinegar and lots of chopped fresh basil. Serve immediately or marinate at room temperature for 1 hour. *Serves 4.*

THE BIG CHILL

Here's how to have your family or guests raving about your green salad. Prepare your salad bowl with a variety of greens. Place salad and salad forks in the freezer for a few minutes. Your salad will have a refreshing crisp texture. Remember, it's only for a few minutes since salad greens wilt if they're frozen.

PER SERVING

Calories: 51

Protein: 1 g

Fat: 2 g

Carbohydrate: 8 g

Fiber: 2 g

Good source: Vitamin C

OLIVE OIL: HEART AND SOUL

Why are we all swooning over olive oil and giving extra virgin olive oil the status of vintage wines? Seductive robust taste is one reason; olive oil's association with a reduced risk of heart disease and breast cancer is another. So drizzle olive oil over pasta where the cream used to go, and enjoy a meal that's good for the heart and soul.

Olive oil is rich in monounsaturated fats, low in saturated fats and a source of the important antioxidant vitamin E. Substituting foods high in monounsaturated fats, such as olive oil, for foods high in saturated fats, such as butter or shortening, can reduce levels of harmful cholesterol in the bloodstream, while leaving the good cholesterol intact — in some cases increasing it. High-fat diets have been associated with heart disease and some cancers, but when dietary fat is primarily monounsaturated, this association seems to be reduced. Populations that consume olive oil as their major source of dietary fat are among the healthiest on earth.

CHOOSING

Waving her spatula authoritatively, a cooking-show host recently decreed, "If you want to save calories, buy light olive oil." Wrong! With such baffled "experts," it's not surprising that there is confusion about olive oil.

A stroll down supermarket aisles will reveal three basic kinds of olive oil. All have about 124 calories and 14 g fat per tablespoon. They are:

Light olive oil:
This is a blend of olive oils so refined that it is almost tasteless. The "light" refers to the flavor, not the calories! It is very pale in color. Use it in recipes where you don't want an olive taste, such as biscotti, coleslaw or a stir-fry.

Olive oil:
A blend of refined olive oils is mixed with some extra virgin olive oil to restore the flavor lost in the refining process. With a taste redolent of olives and a golden color, this is the everyday oil of people in Mediterranean countries. Use it for cooking.

Extra virgin olive oil:
This is the finest olive oil, obtained from the first cold pressing of olives. Fruity and flavorful, often with a deep green-gold or even emerald hue, this oil often commands premium prices. Use it in dishes where a robust olive taste is important, such as salads and pastas, and for dipping bread.

USING

When you want to taste the full, delicate flavor of any olive oil, add it to cooked dishes in the final stages. Select the oil based on your own taste preferences. For example, light and delicate dishes such as fish or soups may be better served by a milder, less fruity olive oil. Heartier, more robust dishes made with red meat and tomato-based sauces may be better with a fruitier, more flavorful olive oil.

STORING OLIVE OIL

If you buy more oil than you can use in a couple of months, pour small quantities into opaque bottles for daily use. Store the rest, sealed in its original container, in the refrigerator for up to 1 year.

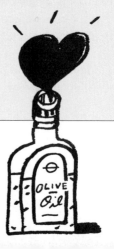

Great Grilling

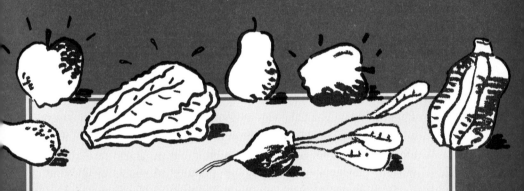

Succulent Grilled Pork Tenderloin with Apples and Leeks

Grilled Portobello Mushroom Salad

Greek Lamb Chops

Asian Barbecued Beef and Greens

Maple-Orange Grilled Chicken with Fruit and Veggies

Lemon Garlic Cornish Hens with Grilled Sweet Peppers
and Polenta

Grilled Seabass with Basil-Lime Marinade

Margarita Salmon Steak

Salsa-Style Mussels on the Grill

Succulent Grilled Pork Tenderloin with Apples and Leeks

We first tasted this sauce on ribs cooked by chef Mark Whalen of the Delawana Inn at the Ducane Barbecue Contest. It was so finger-lickin' good we used it on lean pork tenderloin and added leeks and apples to round out dinner.

PREPARATION TIME: 15 MINUTES / GRILLING TIME: 15 MINUTES

MAKES: 4 TO 6 SERVINGS

2 pork tenderloins, about ¾ lb (375 g) each
¼ cup maple syrup
2 tbsp Dijon mustard
2 tbsp soy sauce
1 tbsp olive oil
2 tsp dried rosemary
2 crushed garlic cloves
¼ tsp maple extract (optional)
4 apples
8 thin leeks

1. Trim any fat from tenderloins. In a small bowl, whisk maple syrup with Dijon, soy and oil. Measure out rosemary and coarsely chop. Add it to mixture along with garlic and maple extract.

2. Slice unpeeled apples in half and core. Trim top third of dark green leaves from leeks. Slice leeks lengthwise through the top green portion but leave at least 2 inches of the white base intact.

3. Oil grill and preheat barbecue to medium. Generously brush marinade over pork tenderloins and place on grill. Close barbecue lid or cover with a tent of foil and grill over medium heat until pork feels slightly springy, about 15 minutes. Turn meat often and brush with marinade. Remove meat from grill and let stand, covered, for 5 minutes before slicing.

BARBECUED SQUASH

To make it easier to slice a hard acorn squash, first make a small slit in the squash, then microwave on high for 2 minutes. Slice into ½-inch rounds. Remove seeds. Brush with olive oil or melted butter. Barbecue with the lid down until squash is tender, about 10 minutes. Turn often.

PER SERVING

Calories: 305

Protein: 26 g

Fat: 7 g

Carbohydrate: 36 g

Fiber: 4 g

Excellent source: Iron

Good source: Folic Acid

---

4. As soon as pork has been put on the grill, lightly brush apples with maple marinade and leeks with oil. Place on grill. Turn them several times as they cook. As soon as apples are hot and grill marks have appeared, and leeks are slightly charred on outside, remove them from grill. Apples will need about 5 to 7 minutes and leeks about 8 to 10 minutes. Peel charred outer leaves from leeks. Serve with sliced pork.

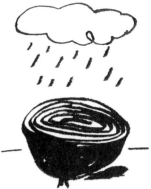

RED ONION

Grilled Portobello Mushroom Salad

Smoky and tender-crisp from grilling, this barbecued vegetable mélange will seduce even those who routinely shun veggies.

PREPARATION TIME: 15 MINUTES / GRILLING TIME: 20 MINUTES

MAKES: 6 ONE-CUP SERVINGS

3 sweet peppers, preferably 1 each of red, green and yellow

10 large portobello mushrooms, about 2 inches in diameter

2 large zucchini, about 6 inches long

1 large onion, preferably red, Vidalia or Spanish

2 tbsp olive oil

2 to 3 tbsp balsamic vinegar

2 crushed garlic cloves

¾ tsp chopped fresh rosemary, ¼ tsp crushed dried rosemary, or 1 tsp dried basil

¾ tsp finely chopped fresh thyme, pinch of dried leaf thyme, or ½ tsp dried leaf oregano

½ tsp salt

¼ tsp freshly ground black pepper

½ cup black or green olives (optional)

2 tomatoes, chopped (optional)

1½ tsp granulated sugar

SWEET GRILLED PARSNIPS

Peel parsnips and slice in half. Brush with olive oil, sesame oil or melted butter. Barbecue with the lid down until golden and as soft as you like, about 5 to 8 minutes per side. Parsnips are great with barbecued pork chops and chicken.

PER SERVING

Calories: 171	
Protein: 8 g	
Fat: 6 g	
Carbohydrate: 28 g	
Fiber: 10 g	

Excellent source: Vitamin C, Folic Acid, Iron

Good source: Vitamin A

1. Preheat barbecue and lightly oil grill. Cut peppers into quarters and seed. Wipe mushrooms with paper towels. Cut zucchini, lengthwise, into ¼-inch slices. Cut onion into 1-inch slices. Stir oil with 2 tablespoons vinegar, garlic, fresh or dried herbs, salt and black pepper.

2. Lightly brush prepared vegetables with dressing. Grill until they are tender-crisp, about 10 minutes for zucchini and mushrooms, 13 minutes for peppers and 20 minutes for onion. Brush occasionally with dressing. Remove vegetables from grill as they are done.

3. Cut hot grilled vegetables into bite-size pieces. Put them in a large mixing bowl with olives and tomatoes. Drizzle with remaining dressing and gently toss. Taste and add more fresh or dried herbs, vinegar and sugar, if needed. Serve warm. Salad will keep well, covered, in the refrigerator, for up to 2 days.

GREAT PASTA SAUCE: *Warm leftovers in a frying pan or microwave. Add a little tomato sauce, if you like, and toss with hot pasta.*

NEW THREE-BEAN SALAD

Mix 19 oz (540 mL) kidney beans, 19 oz (540 mL) Romano beans, 14 oz (398 mL) pinto beans with ½ small chopped red onion, 1 chopped red pepper, ¼ cup Italian dressing and ½ teaspoon each of ground cumin and coriander. *Makes 6 cups.*

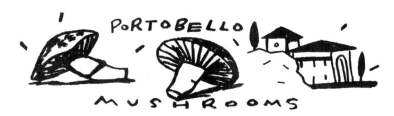

PORTOBELLO MUSHROOMS

Despite their Italian names, portobello and cremini are strains of the familiar white button mushrooms developed in North America. Choose them at their freshest when they're plump and slightly dry to the touch, without wet patches or wrinkling. Because of their large size and meaty texture, portobello mushrooms are the "steak" of the vegetable world. Ideal for grilling, a single mushroom can measure 3 inches or more in diameter, which means it won't slip through the grill. Portobello stems are woody and best reserved for making stock, or discarded. Young robust portobellos (sold as brown or cremini mushrooms), measuring just about 1 inch in diameter, are perfect for stuffing. To clean and prepare, wipe with a clean tea towel or a paper towel; if the gills on the mushroom underside seem sandy, brush lightly to remove grit or rinse very quickly. Do not soak — sponge-like mushrooms absorb water very easily. Store, lightly wrapped in waxed paper or in a brown paper bag, in the crisper section of the refrigerator.

Greek Lamb Chops

Juicy garlicky lamb chops, hot off the grill, are one of the barbecuer's greatest pleasures. We've also added some jazzy complementary vegetables.

PREPARATION TIME: 10 MINUTES / MARINATING TIME: 4 HOURS
GRILLING TIME: 10 MINUTES / MAKES: 4 SERVINGS

8 lamb chops, about ¾ inch thick

2 cups white wine

2 tbsp olive oil

4 crushed garlic cloves

¼ cup chopped fresh oregano or 2 tsp dried leaf oregano

½ tsp salt

½ tsp freshly ground black pepper

4 zucchini

4 ripe but firm tomatoes

1. To avoid flare-ups, trim fat on chops to about ⅛ inch. Stir wine with oil, garlic, oregano, salt and pepper. Put chops in a resealable plastic bag or dish just large enough to hold them in a single layer. Add wine mixture and seal bag or cover dish. Marinate in the refrigerator for at least 4 hours or overnight. If using thawed frozen chops, marinate them overnight. Turn chops 2 or 3 times during marinating time.

2. When ready to cook chops, preheat barbecue and lightly oil grill. Slice zucchini, lengthwise, in half or thirds. Slice tomatoes in half. Drain chops, reserving marinade. Grill chops, basting occasionally with marinade, for about 5 to 6 minutes per side for medium-rare. Baste vegetables with marinade and grill them alongside lamb chops. Zucchini and tomatoes will need about 4 to 5 minutes per side. Baste meat and vegetables occasionally with marinade.

CORN-OFF-THE-COB TOSSED SALAD

Slice kernels from 2 cooked cobs of corn. Mix about 1½ cups kernels with 1 chopped sweet pepper, 2 sliced green onions and ¼ cup Italian dressing. *Makes 2 cups.*

PER SERVING

Calories: 204

Protein: 20 g

Fat: 7 g

Carbohydrate: 12 g

Fiber: 4 g

Good source: Vitamin A, Vitamin C, Folic Acid, Iron

Asian Barbecued Beef and Greens

Here's a healthy entrée that capitalizes on lean steak, ginger and other assertive flavors from Thailand. For a marinade with only 3 ingredients, this one gives amazing flavor. It's also a marvelous tenderizer for an economical steak such as bottom round.

PREPARATION TIME: 10 MINUTES / MARINATING TIME: 3 HOURS

GRILLING TIME: 6 MINUTES / MAKES: 4 TO 6 SERVINGS

---

2 lbs (1 kg) steak such as bottom round, top sirloin, flank steak or eye-of-round roast
¼ cup chili garlic sauce or Sambal Oelek
¼ cup fish sauce
1½ tbsp dark sesame oil
1 tbsp grated or ground fresh ginger or bottled minced ginger (optional)
3 crushed garlic cloves
6 thin green onions
1 small bok choy
3 green peppers
1 lime, cut in half (optional)
¼ to ½ cup chopped fresh coriander (optional)

1. Trim fat from steak. If using eye-of-round, slice into steaks at least 1 inch thick. Place steak, folding in half, if necessary, in a resealable plastic bag or dish large enough to hold it snugly. In a small bowl, whisk garlic sauce with fish sauce, 1 tablespoon sesame oil, ginger and garlic. Pour over steak so meat is evenly coated. Seal bag or cover with plastic wrap. Refrigerate at least 3 hours, preferably overnight, turning bag once.

2. When ready to barbecue, oil grill and preheat barbecue. Prepare vegetables by trimming any tough green leaves from green onions and trim off root ends. Wash bok choy and slice in half lengthwise through stem ends. Remove stem ends from peppers. Slice peppers in half lengthwise and remove seeds.

ORIENTAL CARROT SLAW

Stir 2 cups shredded or grated carrot with 2 tablespoons peanut sauce. Then add ¼ cup chopped fresh coriander. Refrigerate at least until chilled or up to 2 days. *Makes 2 cups.*

PER SERVING

Calories: 244

Protein: 30 g

Fat: 11 g

Carbohydrate: 6 g

Fiber: 2 g

Excellent source: Vitamin C

Good source: Iron

3. Drain marinade from meat into a small dish. Place steak over hottest part of barbecue. Lightly brush peppers with marinade, onions and bok choy with sesame oil, and place them on grill. Turn often, until they are lightly charred, then remove to a cutting board. Meanwhile, brush meat frequently with marinade, until seared and browned, 5 to 6 minutes for medium-rare. Flank steak cooked beyond medium tends to be tough. Remove steak to a cutting board. Immediately squeeze lime juice over top and let steak sit 5 minutes.

4. Thinly slice meat across the grain. The vegetables are terrific sliced and tossed with hot rice as well as any remaining marinade and lots of chopped coriander. The steak is also delicious cut into strips, slathered with sour cream and wrapped in warm tortillas.

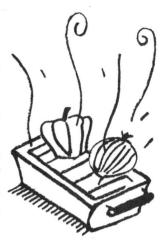

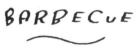

GRILL OVERS

When barbecuing, toss more on the grill than you'll need for supper. Refrigerate extras as soon as they're off the grill. Here are a few delicious ways to enjoy them:

- Cold, thinly sliced grilled steak is wonderful tossed in a Caesar salad or added to a tomato sandwich.

- Freeze grilled burgers. Defrost and heat in the microwave for a 2-minute dinner or healthy snack.

- Grill tomato halves and refrigerate or freeze. For a roasted tomato soup, whirl in a food processor with garlic.

- Barbecue extra fish, seafood and onion slices. Serve in a tomato broth the following day for an outstanding fish soup.

- Grill extra ribs. Freeze. Reheat in a microwave or hot oven. Slice into single ribs for a hearty appetizer.

- Barbecue lots of vegetables. Slice hot veggies into bite-size pieces. Toss with garlicky olive oil, balsamic vinegar and chopped fresh basil. Refrigerate and serve cold as a salad.

- Stir strips of grilled chicken, steak or sausage into store-bought potato or pasta salad for a quick creamy main-course salad.

- For a fast homemade pasta salad, toss coarsely chopped grilled vegetables with hot cooked rotini or penne and your favorite Italian dressing. Serve at room temperature with a grating of Parmesan cheese and a sprinkling of sliced olives or chopped fresh herbs.

- Shred grilled chicken or steak, or crumble burgers. Roll up in flour tortillas along with grated cheese and a slathering of salsa. Serve cold or wrap in waxed paper and heat in the microwave until warm and cheese is gooey.

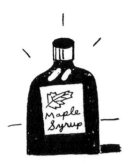

CANADIAN

Maple-Orange Grilled Chicken with Fruit and Veggies

Our winning orange juice and maple syrup baste combo is finger-licking great. Grill everything together on the barbie. P.S. No pans to clean.

PREPARATION TIME: 15 MINUTES / GRILLING TIME: 15 MINUTES
MAKES: 6 TO 8 SERVINGS

PER SERVING OF CHICKEN, FRUIT AND VEGETABLES

Calories: 206

Protein: 28 g

Fat: 2 g

Carbohydrate: 20 g

Fiber: 3 g

Excellent source: Vitamin C

8 skinless boneless chicken breasts

4 medium zucchini

2 peppers, red or green

1 mango or pineapple

2 oranges

⅓ cup frozen orange juice concentrate, undiluted

⅓ cup maple syrup

2 tbsp finely chopped fresh basil or 1 tsp dried basil

GREAT GRILLED VEGGIES

Vegetable	Preparation	Grilling Time	Flavor Boosts
CORN ON THE COB	Wrap in foil.	20 to 25 minutes, turning often.	Butter seasoned with crushed red pepper, cayenne or cumin.
EGGPLANT SLICES	Slice lengthwise. Sprinkle with salt and brush with olive oil.	12 to 15 minutes, turning often.	Garlic- or herb-flavored oil. Top with fresh tomato salsa.
MUSHROOMS	Thread on skewers. Brush with olive oil or melted butter.	4 to 7 minutes, turning often.	Sprinkle with dill, rosemary or chives.
PEPPERS	Slice into halves or quarters. Seed. Brush with oil.	15 to 20 minutes, turning often. Or, cook until charred, then peel.	Brush with garlic oil. Spritz with balsamic vinegar.
ZUCCHINI	Slice lengthwise. Brush with oil or butter.	4 to 6 minutes, turning often.	Brush with garlic butter mixed with basil, tarragon or curry powder.

1. Oil grill and preheat barbecue. Trim any fat from chicken. Diagonally slice zucchini into ¼-inch pieces. Cut peppers into quarters, then remove core and seeds. Peel and slice mango as thickly as possible. Or peel, core and slice pineapple into ½-inch slices. Cut unpeeled oranges into ½-inch slices. Stir orange juice concentrate with maple syrup and basil.

2. Brush sauce over chicken and peppers. Place them on grill. Barbecue until underside of chicken is golden, about 8 to 10 minutes. Turn chicken and peppers, then brush again with sauce. Add zucchini, mango and oranges to grill. Brush with sauce. Continue cooking until chicken is golden and feels springy to the touch, and fruit and vegetables are hot. This will take about 6 to 10 more minutes. Turn zucchini and fruit at least once. Covered and refrigerated, chicken, vegetables and mango will keep well for 1 day. Oranges, however, are best served the day they are grilled.

SUCCULENT INSTEAD OF SINGED BARBECUED CHICKEN

Burning chicken on the barbecue seems to be a universal problem. The intense barbecue heat sears the chicken, but it takes a long time for the heat to cook through to the bones whether you're doing pieces or halves. To prevent burnt birds, microwave chicken until almost cooked, then baste with olive oil or barbecue sauce and grill for 10 to 15 minutes. Always keep the barbecue lid down or cover with a tent of foil.

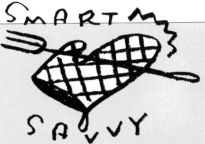

BARBECUE SAVVY

SMART BARBECUING TIPS
- For a smoky flavor, sprinkle 1 cup moistened hickory flakes over hot coals just before putting ribs, chops or fish on grill.
- Cook most foods about 4 inches from the coals. Move larger items further away.
- To ensure even cooking, bring steaks, chops or roasts to room temperature before grilling.

PERFECT STEAK
- To prevent flare-ups, trim all visible fat before grilling.
- To prevent curling, nick outside edges of steak at 2-inch intervals.
- Turn meat with tongs to avoid losing precious juices.
- Press steak with your finger. If steak is soft, it's rare; if steak bounces back, it's medium; if steak feels firm, it's well done.

GRILLING PERFECTION
- Partially cook chicken pieces, pork chops and potatoes in the microwave, then finish on grill.
- For tender grilled ribs, precook in gently boiling water until fork-tender. This may take up to 1 hour. Barbecue right away or refrigerate for up to 2 days. Coat with sauce and grill, turning and basting often, until hot and richly glazed, about 10 to 15 minutes.
- Place a foil drip pan on the coals directly under a large roast or whole chicken.
- To turn delicate fish, place fish steaks in an oiled fish barbecue basket. Or, loosely wrap whole fish in oiled chicken wire.

Lemon Garlic Cornish Hens with Grilled Sweet Peppers and Polenta

When it's barbecue time, you want the cookin' easy. So we designed a fancy yet no-fuss menu starring little golden hens, or chicken pieces if you like, thick slices of polenta and peppers — they all fit on the grill together so everything is ready at the same time.

PREPARATION TIME: 20 MINUTES / GRILLING TIME: 55 MINUTES
MAKES: 2 TO 4 SERVINGS

2 Rock Cornish game hens, about 1½ lbs (750 g) each or 1 chicken

2 lemons

6 crushed garlic cloves, or 1½ tbsp bottled minced garlic

2 tsp hot pepper sauce

½ (1-lb/500-g) roll of ready-to-heat polenta*

2 tbsp olive oil

Grated Parmesan or Romano cheese (optional)

2 large peppers, different colors

1 tbsp balsamic vinegar

Pinches of paprika, salt and pepper

1. If Cornish hens are frozen, thaw them completely. Split in half along the back and breastbone. Or slice chicken into 4 pieces. Finely grate peel from lemons and squeeze out juice. Stir juice and peel with garlic and hot pepper sauce.

2. To precook hens on the barbecue, begin by placing each half, bone-side down, on a piece of heavy foil, large enough to overlap the ends. Bend up sides of foil slightly and pour lemon mixture over top. Tightly seal packets. Place on preheated barbecue, seam-side up, for 25 minutes. Don't turn the packet during this time. Open one end of each packet and pour juices into a heat-proof dish, then unwrap the packet fully.

HONEY GRILLED PEARS

Choose ripe pears. Slice in half. Baste with orange or apple juice sweetened with a little liquid honey. Place pears on a greased grill and cook, basting and turning often, until pears take on a golden hue, about 5 to 8 minutes. Serve warm pears with cambozola cheese or drizzled with yogurt.

PER SERVING

Calories: 521	
Protein: 47	
Fat: 30 g	
Carbohydrate: 15 g	
Fiber: 2 g	
Excellent source: Vitamin A, Vitamin C	
Good source: Iron	

3. Or, to precook hens in the microwave, snugly place halves, skin-side down, in a microwave-safe dish such as an 8-inch (2-L) square dish. Pour lemon mixture over top. Cover and microwave on high for 20 minutes. Save juices. (If making ahead, refrigerate at this point, up to 1 day.)

4. To give a barbecue flavor, place precooked halves on grill, bone-side down. Grill on medium heat, turning often and basting with juices, until golden and meat feels springy, about 30 minutes.

5. As soon as hens are precooking, slice polenta into ½- to 1-inch rounds. Thinner slices will be crispier. Brush all cut surfaces with oil. Place polenta on oiled grill along with the foil packets of Cornish hens, or at the same time you place hens in the microwave. Grill, checking underside occasionally, until golden-tinged and hot, about 15 to 20 minutes per side. If polenta is ready before hens are, move pieces to a cooler part of barbecue or keep warm, uncovered, in the oven. Sprinkle with Parmesan cheese, if you like.

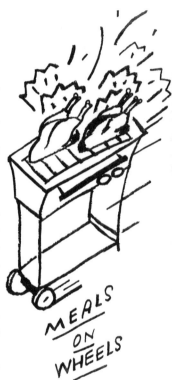

6. After polenta is put on grill, remove stems from peppers and cut peppers into quarters. Remove seeds and white ribs. Stir 1 tablespoon oil with vinegar and seasonings. Brush mixture over pepper wedges. When Cornish hens have been turned skin-side down for their final browning, place peppers on barbecue. Grill, brushing with oil mixture occasionally, until hot and singed around the edges, about 6 minutes per side. Remove from the grill and toss them with any remaining balsamic mixture. Serve hot Cornish hens with peppers and polenta on the side.

SHOPPING TIP: Polenta is now sold in fully prepared rolls in many supermarkets and doesn't need to be refrigerated until opened.

Grilled Seabass with Basil-Lime Marinade

For the most succulent, delicately herbed fish you can imagine, marinate seabass, swordfish or tuna steaks in a fresh basil sauce with Mediterranean overtones. Grill colorful vegetables at the same time.

PREPARATION TIME: 15 MINUTES / MARINATING TIME: 4 HOURS
GRILLING TIME: 12 MINUTES / MAKES: 4 TO 6 SERVINGS

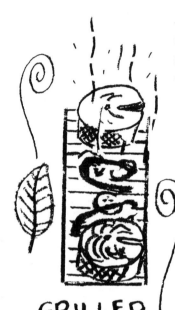

GRILLED SEA BASS

1 large Spanish or red onion, peeled
Juice of 2 limes
2 tbsp olive oil
2 tsp ground paprika or cumin
½ tsp each of cayenne pepper and salt
1 cup loosely packed large basil or coriander leaves
2 lbs (1 kg) seabass fillets or firm-fleshed fish steaks, at least 1 inch thick
2 zucchini
4 peppers, preferably a mix of colors

1. Cut onion into eighths. Place onions in a food processor along with lime juice, oil, seasonings and basil. Whirl, using an on-and-off motion until onions are minced, stopping and scraping down sides.

2. Slice fish fillets into serving-size pieces. Put in a resealable plastic bag. Pour marinade over top. Coat fish evenly. Seal bag and put in a bowl in refrigerator. Marinate at least 4 hours, or overnight. Turn bag occasionally.

3. To barbecue, oil grill and preheat to medium-high. Slice zucchini lengthwise into halves or thirds. Slice peppers into thirds and seed. Brush vegetables with olive oil and place on grill. Remove fish from marinade, leaving most of marinade in bag. Grill fish on barbecue 5 to 6 minutes per side, basting often with marinade. Zucchini will need 5 minutes and peppers about 8 minutes per side. Slice hot vegetables into bite-size pieces. Stir into hot couscous or rice along with lots of sliced green onions and serve beside fish.

PER SERVING

Calories: 268

Protein: 32 g

Fat: 10 g

Carbohydrate: 13 g

Fiber: 3 g

Excellent source: Vitamin C

Good source: Vitamin A, Folic Acid

Margarita Salmon Steak

We got the idea for this recipe from Jane Bailey, a British Columbia cooking teacher. Salmon steaks are marinated in lime, tequila and jalapeños for Mexican kick in this superbly different yet decadent treatment of moist steaks — cha, cha, cha!

PREPARATION TIME: 10 MINUTES / MARINATING TIME: 1 HOUR
GRILLING TIME: 15 MINUTES / MAKES: 4 SERVINGS

3 limes

⅓ cup tequila or vodka

2 tbsp olive oil

2 jalapeño peppers, or 1 tsp hot red pepper flakes

2 tbsp granulated sugar

½ tsp salt

4 salmon steaks, about 1½ inches thick,
  or a 1½-lb (750-g) salmon fillet

Red Pepper Salsa (see recipe at right)

1. Grate peel from limes and place peel in a bowl. Squeeze juice from limes. Add about ½ cup lime juice to the peel along with tequila and oil. Core jalapeño peppers. Remove seeds and discard them. Finely chop peppers and stir into lime mixture with sugar and salt until sugar is dissolved.

2. Put salmon steaks in a large resealable bag or in a dish just large enough to snugly hold them. To support the bag while you fill it, place it in a large bowl, then pour marinade over fish and seal bag. Or pour marinade over salmon and cover dish tightly with plastic wrap. Refrigerate at least 4 hours, preferably overnight.

3. To barbecue, lightly oil grill and set barbecue to medium. Remove salmon from marinade and place salmon directly on the hot grill. Barbecue with the lid closed for about 7 to 8 minutes per side or until the point of a knife inserted in center of the salmon comes out warm. Salmon can also be cooked under the broiler for the same time or baked, uncovered, at 425°F (220°C) for about 15 minutes.

RED PEPPER SALSA
Stir 2 finely chopped red peppers with 2 finely chopped jalapeño peppers. Chop ½ English cucumber and finely chop ½ red onion and add along with 4 sliced green onions. Stir the juice of 2 limes with 2 tablespoons granulated sugar and 2 large crushed garlic cloves. Stir into the salsa vegetables until they are evenly coated. Let sit at room temperature for at least an hour or refrigerate for at least 4 hours. Serve the same day it is made. *Makes 3 cups.*

PER SALMON STEAK WITH SALSA

Calories: 322

Protein: 31 g

Fat: 17 g

Carbohydrate: 10 g

Fiber: Trace

Good source: Vitamin C, Folic Acid

4. While salmon is grilling, pour remaining marinade into a saucepan. Boil vigorously, uncovered and stirring often, until sauce is reduced by at least half. This will take about 3 minutes of boiling. Pour over hot salmon steaks. Serve with Red Pepper Salsa.

Salsa-Style Mussels on the Grill

Yes, mussels can be cooked on the barbecue. Here's a delicious and inexpensive appetizer for four or dinner for two.

PREPARATION TIME: 15 MINUTES / GRILLING TIME: 15 MINUTES

MAKES: 2 MAIN COURSES OR 4 APPETIZERS

3 lbs (1.5 kg) fresh mussels
½ cup dry white wine
1½ tsp olive oil
2 crushed garlic cloves
2 firm tomatoes, seeded and chopped
2 green onions, thinly sliced
1 banana or 2 jalapeño peppers, seeded and finely chopped

1. Scrub mussels under cold running water and remove any beards. Discard any mussels that are open and will not close when gently tapped. Drain mussels well. Place them in a large foil lasagna pan or other large, shallow metal pan that will fit on the barbecue, such as a 9 x 13-inch (3-L) pan. Stir wine with oil and garlic. Pour mixture over mussels. Sprinkle with tomatoes, green onions and peppers. Cover pan tightly with foil. Cook right away or refrigerate for up to 6 hours.

2. Place sealed foil pan on preheated barbecue. Cook until foil over pan is hot and domed, about 15 minutes, or 18 minutes if pan has been refrigerated. Mussels should be open and broth hot. Discard any mussels that have not opened. Serve right away from foil pan or in heated serving bowls. Dip crusty bread into broth.

TOMATOES

Tomatoes get their bright red color from lycopene, an important antioxidant, which has shown promise in reducing the risk of prostate and colon cancers. Tomatoes are also rich in vitamin C, potassium and beta-carotene. One whole tomato contains about 26 calories.

PER MAIN-COURSE SERVING

Calories: 222

Protein: 21 g

Fat: 7 g

Carbohydrate: 14 g

Fiber: 2 g

Excellent source: Vitamin A, Vitamin C, Folic Acid, Iron

Oodles of Noodles

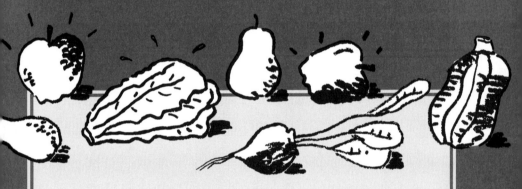

Moroccan Saffron Tomato Sauce

Linguine with Roasted Red Peppers and Smoked Chicken

Thai Chicken Noodle Salad

Shanghai Noodle Salad

Singapore Curried Shrimp and Noodles

New-Style Pad Thai

Freezer-Friendly Spaghetti Sauce

Easy-Make, Easy-Eat Layered Pasta Bake

Moroccan Saffron Tomato Sauce

This appealing saffron-laced sauce is the signature of Charles Obadia of the Boujadi Moroccan Restaurant in Toronto. We've simplified the cooking but managed to create most of the same flavor. Spoon this big-batch sauce over chicken or fish on a bed of couscous. We love it tossed with pasta and shrimp.

PREPARATION TIME: 30 MINUTES
COOKING TIME: 1 HOUR AND 40 MINUTES / MAKES: 18 CUPS

2 to 4 tbsp olive oil
4 onions, peeled and coarsely chopped
10 crushed garlic cloves
4 peppers, preferably 2 red and 2 green
10 large fresh tomatoes, about 3 lbs (1.5 kg)
2 (28-oz/796-mL) cans plum tomatoes
2 tbsp paprika
1½ to 3 tsp hot red pepper flakes
1 tsp saffron threads
¼ tsp turmeric
½ tsp salt
¼ to ½ tsp cayenne pepper
14-oz (398-mL) can tomato sauce
5½-oz (156-mL) can tomato paste
1 cup chopped fresh coriander

1. Heat oil in a large saucepan set over medium heat. Add onions and garlic and sauté, stirring often, until soft, at least 10 minutes. Meanwhile, seed and chop peppers. Peel tomatoes only if you wish and coarsely chop. When onions are soft, add tomatoes and any juices, peppers, canned tomatoes with juice, seasonings, tomato sauce and paste. Bring to a boil. Reduce heat to low, cover and simmer for 1½ hours, stirring often. Add coriander for the last 10 minutes of cooking. Serve right away, refrigerate up to 4 days or freeze up to 4 months.

ONION SAVVY

If you have lots of onions to chop, wear goggles or burn a candle beside chopping board. Onion odors on your hands? Rub them briskly with salt before washing. To avoid onion breath, eat a few sprigs of parsley.

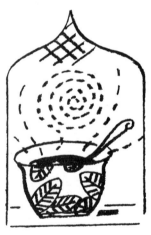

PER CUP

Calories: 87

Protein: 3 g

Fat: 2 g

Carbohydrate: 17 g

Fiber: 4 g

Excellent source: Vitamin A, Vitamin C

Linguine with Roasted Red Peppers and Smoked Chicken

A simple sauce gets smoky flavor from deli chicken and freshly roasted peppers (buy a jar to save time). And this pasta dinner is not only lower in fat, it's also a really good source of iron.

PREPARATION TIME: 20 MINUTES / COOKING TIME: 15 MINUTES

MAKES: 4 SERVINGS

10-oz (313-mL) jar roasted red peppers, or 4 red peppers, roasted

2 tbsp olive oil

2 crushed garlic cloves

½ lb (250 g) mushrooms, sliced

¾ tsp salt

½ tsp sugar

Pinch of cayenne pepper

½ (1-lb/450-g) pkg dry linguine or fettuccine

2 cups coarsely chopped, deli-smoked or cooked chicken

2 green onions, thinly sliced

1. Purée peppers, including juice, in a food processor or blender. Bring a pot of salted water to a full rolling boil. Heat oil in a frying pan set over medium-high heat. Add garlic, mushrooms, salt, sugar and cayenne to oil in pan. Sauté mushrooms, stirring frequently, until they lose most of their moisture, about 5 minutes.

2. Add pasta to boiling water. Stir to separate and boil until al dente, about 8 minutes. Stir chicken and puréed red pepper into mushrooms. When mixture is hot, toss it with hot drained pasta and green onions. Serve immediately sprinkled with grated Parmesan cheese.

FOR VEGETARIANS: *In place of adding chicken with the pepper purée, add about a half cup of creamy crumbled chèvre or grated smoked cheese or Asiago.*

ROASTED PEPPERS

Preheat broiler. Broil peppers 4 inches from heat, turning frequently, until blackened on all sides. To soften skin, place peppers in a paper or plastic bag. Seal and leave about 5 minutes. Peel off skin and seed, saving all juices. Store covered in the refrigerator for up to 2 days or freeze.

PER SERVING

Calories:	347
Protein:	26 g
Fat:	13 g
Carbohydrate:	32 g
Fiber:	4 g
Excellent source:	Vitamin A, Vitamin C
Good source:	Folic Acid, Iron

Thai Chicken Noodle Salad

East meets West in this lively blend of flavors. You'll discover, as we did, that "reduced fat" needn't mean boring! This Oriental salad is equally great for a picnic or a formal party.

PREPARATION TIME: 30 MINUTES / COOKING TIME: 20 MINUTES

MAKES: 12 CUPS

1-lb (450-g) pkg spaghetti
2 tsp sesame oil*
3 to 4 limes
2 tbsp soy sauce
2 tsp Sambal Oelek or Oriental chili-garlic sauce*
1 tsp each of salt and sugar
4 skinless boneless chicken breasts
1 red pepper, seeded
2 to 3 carrots
1 onion
4 celery stalks
¼ lb (125 g) snow peas
2 tbsp olive oil
2 crushed garlic cloves
¼ to ½ cup water
¼ to ½ cup finely chopped fresh coriander
4 green onions, thinly sliced

1. Cook pasta according to package directions for minimum time suggested, usually 8 minutes. Drain and rinse with cold water until cool. Drain again. Place in a large bowl and stir with sesame oil. Finely grate peel from 1 lime and squeeze enough juice from limes to measure ¼ cup. Stir juice with peel, soy sauce, Sambal Oelek, salt and sugar. Stir with pasta to coat.

2. Slice chicken into bite-size pieces. Thinly slice pepper and carrots into long strips. Thinly slice onion and celery. Trim ends from snow peas.

PERFECT PASTA

- Use plenty of water — a 6- to 8-quart (6- to 8-L) pot filled two-thirds full is ideal to cook a 1-lb (450-g) package.
- To heighten pasta flavor, add 2 to 3 teaspoons salt to water.
- Bring water to a rolling boil before adding pasta. Add all at once, stirring immediately to keep pieces separated.
- Boil, uncovered, stirring often, over high heat. After the minimum amount of cooking time stated on package, remove 1 piece and bite into it. If it is firm and doesn't have a white uncooked area in the center, it is perfectly cooked!

PER CUP

Calories: 233

Protein: 15 g

Fat: 4 g

Carbohydrate: 33 g

Fiber: 3 g

Excellent source: Vitamin A

Good source: Vitamin C

3. Heat 1 tablespoon olive oil in a large frying pan set over medium-high heat. Add half of chicken and cook, stirring often, until lightly browned, about 3 minutes. Remove chicken from pan. Repeat with remaining oil and chicken. Return chicken and any juices to pan. Add garlic and onion. Cook until onion has softened, about 3 minutes.

4. Stir in ¼ cup water, pepper, celery and carrots. Continue cooking, stirring often, until hot, about 3 minutes, adding more water, 1 tablespoon at a time, to keep a little sauce visible under mixture. Add peas. Stir until they are bright green, about 1 minute. Toss with spaghetti, coriander and green onions. Serve right away. Or, if taking to a picnic, refrigerate, uncovered, until cold or for up to 1 day.

SHOPPING TIP: Sesame oil, Sambal Oelek and chili-garlic sauce are found in supermarkets where soy sauce is sold, as well as in specialty food stores.

Shanghai Noodle Salad

Oriental flavors dominate in this light noodle salad that's a specialty at The Acton Grill in Wolfville, N.S. Let it add a fresh twist to your next buffet.

PREPARATION TIME: 20 MINUTES / COOKING TIME: 10 MINUTES
MAKES: 12 TO 16 SERVINGS

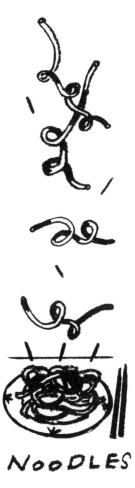

NOODLES

DRESSING

2 tbsp freshly squeezed lime juice, 1 to 2 limes

2 tbsp soy sauce

2 tbsp vegetable oil

1 tbsp brown sugar

2 tsp Sambal Oelek or Oriental chili-garlic sauce

2 tsp sesame oil

1 tbsp grated or finely minced fresh or bottled garlic

3 large crushed garlic cloves

½ tsp salt

PER SERVING	
Calories: 250	
Protein: 9 g	
Fat: 4 g	
Carbohydrate: 44 g	
Fiber: 4 g	
Good source: Vitamin C	

THREE-MINUTE TOMATO PASTA TOSS

Heat 2 tablespoons olive oil and 2 crushed garlic cloves in a large frying pan over medium heat. Add 3 chopped tomatoes, along with any juices, ¼ teaspoon each of salt, pepper and hot pepper sauce. Cook, uncovered and stirring often, until tomatoes begin to soften, about 3 minutes. Meanwhile, plunge ½ (1-lb/500-g) package angel hair pasta into boiling water. Stir until separated. Boil, uncovered, until al dente, about 3 minutes. Meanwhile remove tomatoes from heat. Stir in ½ cup chopped chives or 4 thinly sliced green onions. Drain pasta well and toss with sauce. *Serves 4.*

SALAD

2 lbs (1 kg) fresh Shanghai noodles, or
  3 (12-oz/400-g) pkgs fresh Oriental
  Shanghai Miki noodles*
1 large onion
2 peppers, 1 red and 1 green
1 tsp vegetable oil
4 to 6 green onions (optional)
2 cups cooked roast beef strips (optional)

1. Prepare dressing by whisking all dressing ingredients together. If possible, make a few hours ahead and leave at room temperature or make a day ahead and refrigerate.

2. Prepare noodles according to package directions. (We place them in a colander, then run warm water over them for 4 minutes, separating noodles as soon as they are softened.) Drain well, then put in a large bowl.

3. Slice onion and peppers into thin strips. Heat oil in a frying pan. Add onion and sauté until soft, about 5 minutes. Stir in peppers and sauté for 1 minute. Meanwhile, thinly slice green onions. Toss noodles with onion-and-pepper mixture, green onions, roast beef strips, if using, and dressing until mixed.

MAKE AHEAD: *Salad keeps well for at least 1 day in the refrigerator. Or, prepare several hours ahead and leave at room temperature. Stir in roast beef just before serving.*

SHOPPING TIP: *Many supermarkets now sell fresh Oriental noodles in clear packages in the fresh-produce section. Jars of chili-garlic sauce are sold alongside Oriental sauces.*

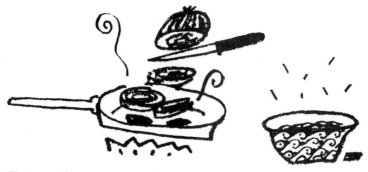

Singapore Curried Shrimp and Noodles

Twelve minutes' cooking time nets you a spicy stir-fry. And it will look and taste like a dish from your favorite Oriental restaurant.

PREPARATION TIME: 20 MINUTES / COOKING TIME: 12 MINUTES
MAKES: 6 SERVINGS

½ (1-lb/500-g) pkg rice-stick noodles
2 skinless boneless chicken breasts
½ lb (250 g) uncooked medium shrimp
1 red pepper
1 tbsp olive oil
1 crushed garlic clove
2 tsp curry powder
Pinch of hot red pepper flakes (optional)
½ cup chicken bouillon or broth
¾ tsp salt
¼ lb (125 g) snow peas, cut in half if large
2 cups bean sprouts
4 green onions, sliced
1 tbsp sesame oil, preferably dark

1. Pour enough boiling water over noodles to cover them. Soak them for 5 minutes, then drain. Rinse with cold water. Slice chicken into bite-size pieces. Shell shrimp and rinse under cold running water. Slice red pepper into julienne strips.

2. Heat olive oil in a nonstick frying pan set over medium-high heat. Stir in garlic and red pepper. Sprinkle mixture with curry powder and red pepper flakes. Stir-fry, adding 1 to 2 tablespoons water to create steam, until pepper is tender-crisp, about 3 minutes.

3. Add chicken and stir-fry for 2 minutes. Add shrimp and stir-fry until it is pink, about 2 minutes. Add bouillon and salt. When mixture is boiling, stir in snow peas, noodles, bean sprouts, onions and sesame oil. Stir-fry until hot. Serve immediately.

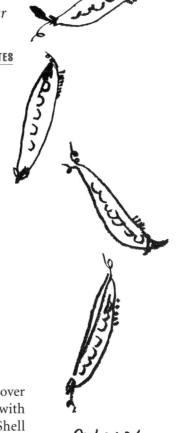

SNOW
PEAS

PER SERVING

Calories:	282
Protein:	20 g
Fat:	6 g
Carbohydrate:	36 g
Fiber:	2 g
Excellent source:	Vitamin C
Good source:	Folic Acid, Iron

New-Style Pad Thai

Pad Thai is one of our longtime food passions. We're always trying to improve on our own recipes. Here's its latest evolution in party-batch size with less fat, more veggies and flavor than we've ever been able to achieve before.

PREPARATION TIME: 45 MINUTES / COOKING TIME: 15 MINUTES

SOAKING TIME: 15 MINUTES / MAKES: 8 SERVINGS

1 lb (400 g) flat rice noodles or rice stick noodles
½ lb (250 g) firm tofu
2 to 3 large skinless boneless chicken breasts
1 lb (500 g) tiger shrimp
3 small peppers, preferably red and yellow
1 tbsp finely chopped garlic
1 bunch coriander
6 thin green onions
4 cups fresh bean sprouts
3 large limes
3 tbsp granulated sugar
¼ cup tamarind sauce
⅓ cup fish sauce
4 tsp hot red chili paste
2 eggs
1 tbsp dried shrimp powder, or ¼ cup dried shrimp
3 tbsp olive oil

RICE NOODLES

Transparent noodles made from ground rice need no cooking. Just cover with boiling water and soak until as soft as you like, about 15 minutes. These noodles are now sold at most supermarkets, as well as in Oriental stores.

1. Rinse noodles with warm water. Place them in a large bowl and cover with warm water. Let soak at room temperature to soften, for at least 15 minutes.

2. Meanwhile, prepare all ingredients before starting to cook. Cut tofu into ½-inch cubes. Slice chicken into thin strips. Cut strips into bite-size lengths. Peel shrimp, leaving tails on if you like. Seed peppers, then slice into thin strips. Finely chop garlic. Wash coriander well and coarsely chop it. Slice green onions. Measure out the bean sprouts.

PER SERVING

Calories: 460

Protein: 31 g

Fat: 11 g

Carbohydrate: 61 g

Fiber: 3 g

Excellent source: Vitamin C, Folic Acid, Iron

Good source: Vitamin A

3. Make the sauce by squeezing the juice from 2 limes and pouring it into a bowl. Stir in sugar, tamarind sauce, fish sauce and hot chili paste. Add eggs and whisk mixture until ingredients are evenly blended. Stir in the dried shrimp powder, or measure out ¼ cup dried shrimp, then finely chop before adding them to the sauce.

4. To cook tofu, pour 1½ tablespoons oil into a large wide saucepan. Place pan over medium-high heat. Add about half the tofu cubes. Sir often and gently with a wide spatula until fairly evenly golden, about 4 minutes. Remove to paper towels to drain. Repeat with remaining tofu, adding more oil if needed.

5. Add 1 tablespoon oil to the pan. Add shrimp and stir often just until pink, about 2 minutes. Do not overcook. Remove shrimp and set aside with the tofu. Add all the chicken and garlic and stir-fry over medium-high heat for 2 minutes, adding more oil if needed. Add all the peppers and stir-fry for 3 minutes. Drain noodles and add them to the pan. Immediately whisk the sauce and pour over noodles. Stir constantly over medium-high heat until noodles are evenly coated. Add the bean sprouts and stir-fry for 3 minutes until noodles are hot. Stir in the tofu, most of the shrimp and any juices, and about half the coriander and green onions. Toss with 2 large wide spatulas. Turn onto a large platter. Scatter the remaining shrimp, coriander and green onions over top. Surround with lime wedges for squeezing over top.

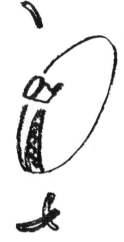

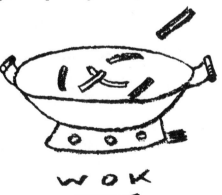

WOK

Freezer-Friendly Spaghetti Sauce

What could be better than a ladleful of homemade spaghetti sauce filled with veggies? Not having to prepare it at the end of the day!

PREPARATION TIME: 25 MINUTES

COOKING TIME: 1 HOUR AND 10 MINUTES / MAKES: 9 TO 12 CUPS

2 tbsp olive oil or other vegetable oil

4 large onions, chopped

4 crushed cloves garlic

2 lbs (1 kg) lean ground beef, or chicken or turkey (optional)

12 large unpeeled tomatoes, coarsely chopped, about 8 cups

14-oz (398-mL) can tomato sauce

5½-oz (156-mL) can tomato paste

2 green peppers, seeded and chopped (optional)

3 chicken bouillon cubes, crushed (optional)

2 bay leaves

2 tsp brown sugar

1 tbsp dried basil, or 1 cup chopped fresh basil

1 tsp dried leaf oregano, or 2 tbsp chopped fresh oregano

1 tsp dried leaf thyme, or 1 tbsp chopped fresh thyme

½ tsp rubbed sage, or 1 tbsp chopped fresh sage

1 tsp hot pepper sauce

1 tsp salt

1. Heat oil in a very large heavy-bottomed saucepan. Add onions, garlic and meat, if using. Cook mixture over medium heat, stirring often until onions are softened, about 5 minutes or until meat loses its pink color. Add remaining ingredients, but if using fresh basil stir in only ½ cup. Bring to a boil, stirring often.

PER CUP
WITHOUT MEAT AND PEPPERS

Calories: 126	
Protein: 4 g	
Fat: 4 g	
Carbohydrate: 23 g	
Fiber: 5 g	
Excellent source: Vitamin A, Vitamin C	
Good source: Iron	

2. Reduce heat to low. Cover and simmer, stirring frequently, for 1 hour to blend flavors. Taste and add more salt or sugar, if you like. Stir in remaining ½ cup fresh basil, if using. Remove bay leaves. Serve tossed with hot pasta or over rice. Covered and refrigerated, it will keep well for 2 days if beef or chicken is added, or at least 4 days if meatless. If frozen, sauce will begin to lose flavor punch after a month or two in the freezer, but will keep well for a year if properly wrapped. After reheating, taste and stir in a little crushed garlic, a sprinkling of herbs, or finely chopped fresh peppers for added texture.

Easy-Make, Easy-Eat Layered Pasta Bake

This multi-layered pasta dinner is a no-fuss vegetarian alternative to lasagna.

PREPARATION TIME: 30 MINUTES / COOKING TIME: 15 MINUTES
BAKING TIME: 35 MINUTES / MAKES: 12 SERVINGS

1-lb (450-g) pkg fettuccine or corkscrew pasta
3 cups spaghetti sauce or a 24-oz (725-mL) container
2 cups salsa, mild or medium
4 crushed cloves garlic
1 large onion
2 green peppers, seeded
2 zucchini
1-lb (475-g) container ricotta cheese, about 2 cups
2 eggs, beaten (optional)
¼ tsp each of nutmeg, salt and pepper
3 cups shredded cheese, such as mozzarella, cheddar or a 4-cheese blend

SPAGHETTI SAUCE PERK-UPS

- Fire up the flavor with a generous sprinkling of hot red pepper flakes or cayenne pepper, dashes of hot pepper sauce or spoonfuls of hot salsa sauce.

- Add a sprinkling of sliced green onions, chopped fresh parsley or coriander. Stir in chopped olives or tomatoes, sliced mushrooms or celery for the last few minutes of simmering.

- Make it fiber-rich by adding lots of diced carrots, broccoli florets and zucchini chunks. Or, serve sauce over spaghetti squash instead of pasta.

- Instead of adding meat, stir cubes of feta, cream cheese or crumbled chèvre into simmering sauce. Or, coarsely grate bits of dried-out or leftover cheese into hot sauce and stir over heat just until soft.

PER SERVING
Calories: 382
Protein: 17 g
Fat: 15 g
Carbohydrate: 46 g
Fiber: 4 g
Excellent source: Vitamin A, Vitamin C, Calcium

SWANKY LINGUINE WITH TEN-MINUTE TOMATO SAUCE

Cook ¾ (1-lb/450-g) package linguine according to package directions. Meanwhile, stir entire contents of 19-oz (540-mL) can Italian-style tomatoes into a wide frying pan set over medium-high heat. Add ¼ cup vermouth or dry red wine and 4 large crushed garlic cloves. Bring to a boil. Continue boiling gently, stirring often, until thickened, about 5 to 7 minutes. Drain cooked linguine and return to cooking pot. Add sauce and cook, stirring often, until pasta is hot, about 2 minutes. Sprinkle with freshly grated Parmesan or Romano. *Serves 3 to 4.*

1. Cook pasta according to package directions for minimum cooking time. When al dente, drain pasta, rinse with cold running water until cool and drain again. Lightly oil two 7 x 11-inch (18 x 28-cm) baking dishes or 2 dishes that can each hold 10 cups (2.5 L). Preheat oven to 350°F (180°C).

2. Pour spaghetti sauce and salsa into a large saucepan set over medium heat. Immediately crush garlic into sauce. Chop onion and add to sauce. Coarsely chop peppers and zucchini. Stir them into sauce. Adjust heat to low and simmer, uncovered, while preparing rest of casserole, at least 10 minutes. Stir often.

3. In a medium-size bowl, stir ricotta cheese with eggs and seasonings until evenly blended. (Eggs will firm ricotta layer.) Set aside 1 cup of grated cheese for top of lasagna. Stir remaining grated cheese into spaghetti sauce, then stir in pasta.

4. Put half of pasta mixture in prepared dishes and gently press down. Evenly spread ricotta mixture over pasta mixture, then top with remaining pasta. Sprinkle with remaining cheese. At this point, casseroles can be baked, or covered and refrigerated for up to 2 days or frozen. If baking right away, place in center of the pre-heated oven and bake, uncovered, until cheese is lightly browned and a knife inserted into center feels warm, about 30 to 35 minutes. If casserole has been refrigerated or frozen, place uncovered cold defrosted casserole in preheated oven and bake until piping hot, about 40 to 55 minutes.

FREEZER SAVVY: *Tightly wrap baked or unbaked casserole and freeze for up to 2 months. Defrost whole baked or unbaked casserole in refrigerator overnight. Bake cold casserole, uncovered, at 350°F (180°C) until piping hot, about 40 to 55 minutes. Check halfway through baking time, and if cheese is becoming too brown before casserole is hot, loosely cover it with a piece of foil.*

For single servings, cut baked casserole into serving-size pieces. Wrap tightly in foil and freeze. Before reheating, remove foil. Place a frozen serving on a microwave-safe plate. Cover with plastic wrap, turning back one corner, or with waxed paper and microwave on medium for 8 to 10 minutes.

Updated Weekday Dinners

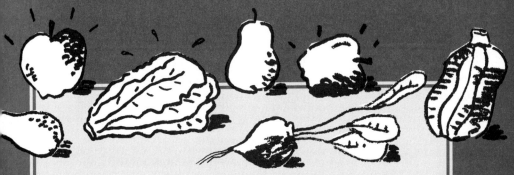

Mediterranean Fish Steaks with Herbed Tomatoes and Olives

Lemon Chicken Dinner with Roasted Garlic

Chicken with Lots of Garlic

Moroccan Chicken with Couscous

Easy Oven-Barbecued Chicken Dinner

Terrific Teriyaki Chicken

Spicy Pork and Peppers

Fast Maple-Mustard Pork Chops and Squash Purée

Grilled Dijon Flank Steak with Spuds and Peppers

New-Style Easy Stuffed Peppers

Couscous with Stir-Fried Spring Vegetables

Vegetarian Mushroom and Red Pepper Cabbage Rolls

Lusty Vegetable Stew with Feta and Basil

Mediterranean Fish Steaks with Herbed Tomatoes and Olives

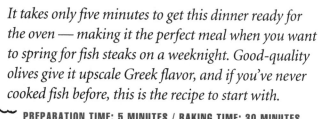

It takes only five minutes to get this dinner ready for the oven — making it the perfect meal when you want to spring for fish steaks on a weeknight. Good-quality olives give it upscale Greek flavor, and if you've never cooked fish before, this is the recipe to start with.

PREPARATION TIME: 5 MINUTES / BAKING TIME: 30 MINUTES
MAKES: 2 TO 3 SERVINGS

PER SERVING

Calories: 220

Protein: 31 g

Fat: 6 g

Carbohydrate: 9 g

Fiber: 2 g

Good source: Vitamin C, Iron

1 tbsp olive oil (optional)

1 lb (500 g) fresh or frozen fish steaks, such as swordfish, tuna or halibut, at least 1 inch thick*

¼ tsp each of salt and freshly ground black pepper

19-oz (540-mL) can Italian-style stewed tomatoes, drained

1 celery stalk, chopped (optional)

2 green onions, thinly sliced

SALMON STEAKS FOR SINGLES

Salmon steak with hollandaise sauce was one of the first fancy fish dishes many of us learned to make. Today, salmon is still considered a treat, but we've learned that its rich taste doesn't need a heavy fat coating. Try these ways to dress up a single salmon steak. For two, simply double the ingredients.

BBQ SALMON WITH CILANTRO SAUCE

Slice a lime in half. Squeeze juice from 1 half over both sides of a salmon steak, then lightly oil it. Grill on a barbecue or broil until a knife point inserted in center of steak comes out warm, about 5 minutes per side.

Meanwhile, prepare sauce by squeezing juice from remaining lime half into a small saucepan. Add ½ cup white wine and ½ teaspoon ground cumin. Boil, uncovered, until reduced to ¼ cup. Stir in ¼ cup chopped fresh cilantro. Pour over salmon.

BAKED SALMON PROVENÇAL

Blend ¼ cup white wine with 1 teaspoon olive oil, 1 large crushed garlic clove, ¼ teaspoon dried leaf thyme and ¼ teaspoon dried tarragon. Pour over salmon and bake in a preheated 450°F (230°C) oven, uncovered and basting often, for 10 minutes.

¼ cup each of small green and black olives (optional)

Generous pinch of cayenne pepper

1. Preheat oven to 450°F (230°C). Pour ½ tablespoon oil into a baking dish that will hold steaks snugly, about 8 x 8 inches (20 x 20 cm). Tip dish so oil coats bottom. Or coat dish with nonstick cooking spray. Season steaks with salt and pepper. (If using frozen fish, simply rinse them with water. Do not defrost them.) Place steaks in dish. Drizzle them with remaining ½ tablespoon oil, if you like.

2. In a small bowl, stir tomatoes with celery, if using, green onions, olives and cayenne. Pour mixture over fish steaks and cover dish with foil. Bake in center of oven until the point of a knife inserted in center of a steak comes out warm, about 30 minutes for fresh fish or up to 50 minutes for frozen. Serve with rice or spiral pasta, and spoon some of tomato sauce over top.

*****FROZEN FISH STEAKS:** *If you use a package of frozen fish steaks, there is no need to defrost them. Simply rinse the steaks with warm water and increase baking time to 40 minutes.*

TEN-MINUTE SOLE DIVAN DINNER

Place 10-oz (280-g) package frozen fish fillets, defrosted, in a single layer, overlapping thin edges, in a shallow baking dish or large pie plate. Lightly spread with 2 teaspoons Dijonnaise or a mix of Dijon mustard and mayonnaise. Arrange 2 cups broccoli florets around outer edge. Cover with plastic wrap, venting one side. Microwave on high for 4 minutes until fish flakes easily with a fork. Drain off juices. Move broccoli to top of fillets. Cover with sliced mozzarella cheese and microwave on high, uncovered, until cheese begins to melt, about 1½ minutes. Serve with rice. *Serves 2.*

WARM SALMON SALAD

Lightly spread top of a salmon steak with Dijon mustard. Sprinkle steak with dried dillweed or chopped fresh dill. Wrap in a packet of foil and seal tightly. Bake in a preheated 450°F (230°C) oven for 20 to 22 minutes. Serve on a bed of mixed spring greens, such as spinach and watercress, that have been tossed with a lemon-vinaigrette dressing.

LEMON-PEPPER SALMON

Stir finely grated peel of half a lemon with juice of 1 whole lemon, ½ teaspoon coarsely ground black pepper and a pinch of ground white pepper. Place 1 salmon steak on a plate. Pour mixture over top. Cover with waxed paper or plastic wrap. Microwave on high until a knife point inserted in center of steak comes out warm, about 1½ to 2 minutes.

SALMON AU POIVRE

Mix 1 tablespoon sherry or port with 1 tablespoon soy sauce and 1 teaspoon brown sugar. Rub into both sides of a salmon steak. Sprinkle both sides with coarsely ground black pepper. Bake, uncovered, in a preheated 450°F (230°C) oven for 10 minutes. Or, sauté in frying pan set over medium-high heat for 3 to 5 minutes per side.

Lemon Chicken Dinner with Roasted Garlic

Roasting garlic tames its assertive flavor, making it almost creamy. Don't let the whole head of garlic deter you from trying this oven dinner with a full-flavored lemony sauce.

PREPARATION TIME: 15 MINUTES / BAKING TIME: 55 MINUTES

MAKES: 6 SERVINGS

1 whole head of garlic
1 lemon
2 tbsp olive oil
½ to 1 cup white wine
1 tbsp honey
½ tsp salt
¼ tsp cayenne pepper
¼ cup finely chopped fresh basil or coriander, or 2 tbsp chopped fresh rosemary, thyme or oregano
6 chicken breasts, bone-in
1 lb (500 g) parsnips or carrots
1 head fennel (optional)
2 lbs (1 kg) small new potatoes
½ cup light sour cream (optional)

1. Preheat oven to 375°F (190°C). Separate garlic head into cloves but do not peel them. Grate peel from lemon and squeeze out 1 tablespoon juice. Put lemon peel and juice in a small dish. Whisk in oil, wine, honey, salt and cayenne until blended. Stir in chopped herbs. Remove skin from chicken. Peel parsnips or carrots and cut into thick long "French fries" about ½ inch thick. Remove stems from fennel and thinly slice the remaining fennel.

SUPERFAST CHICKEN DINNER SOUP

Pour 3 cups chicken broth or bouillon and 1 tablespoon soy sauce into an 8-cup (2-L) microwave-safe bowl. Microwave, covered, on high until boiling, about 5 minutes. Slice 4 skinless chicken breasts into bite-size pieces. Stir in along with ¼ lb (125 g) sliced mushrooms. Microwave, covered, on high until boiling and chicken loses its pink color, about 4 minutes. Stir 3 cups coarsely shredded spinach leaves and 3 green onions into soup. Cover and microwave on medium 2 minutes. *Makes 6 cups.*

PER SERVING

Calories:	347
Protein:	31 g
Fat:	6 g
Carbohydrate:	43 g
Fiber:	5 g
Excellent source:	Folic Acid
Good source:	Vitamin C, Iron

GARLIC

2. Place chicken breasts in a large 11 x 13-inch (3.5-L) broiling pan or divide them between 2 (9 x 13-inch/3-L) baking dishes. Pour lemon mixture over top. Sprinkle with whole garlic cloves. Tuck unpeeled potatoes, parsnips and fennel around chicken. Roast, uncovered, in center of oven for 30 minutes. Turn breasts and baste with pan juices. Add another ½ cup wine, if needed. Continue baking, basting occasionally, until chicken is golden and feels springy, about 25 to 30 more minutes.

3. Remove chicken and vegetables and cover to keep warm. Remove garlic cloves to a small plate. Using a fork, squeeze soft garlic from each clove and discard peel. Mash garlic with fork. Skim any fat from pan juices, then stir in mashed garlic. Whisk in sour cream, if you like. Drizzle over chicken.

Chicken with Lots of Garlic

Chicken with 40 cloves of garlic (yes, it's really 40!), a classic Provençal dish, cooks the garlic long and slowly until sweet and aromatic. Here's a cheater's version Monda does when she gets home from work. It uses only four cloves of garlic and gives the same flavor return with a minimum of fat.

PREPARATION TIME: 10 MINUTES / COOKING TIME: 25 MINUTES

MAKES: 4 SERVINGS

4 skinless boneless chicken breasts

1 tsp butter or olive oil

1 cup white wine

1 chicken bouillon cube

1 tsp each of dried tarragon and Dijon mustard

4 large crushed garlic cloves

2 bunches of spinach or a 10-oz (284-g) bag of spinach

¼ cup light sour cream (optional)

SALMON SUPPER SALAD

Tear 1 bunch spinach or 1 head lettuce into bite-size pieces. Place spinach in a salad bowl along with ¼ unpeeled English cucumber, cut in half lengthwise and thinly sliced, and 2 thinly sliced green onions. Mix 2 tablespoons light mayonnaise with 1 teaspoon soy sauce and ½ teaspoon grated orange peel. Toss dressing with spinach mixture until spinach is evenly coated. Lightly flake a 6½-oz (184-g) can salmon and sprinkle it over top. *Serves 2.*

PER SERVING

Calories: 179

Protein: 30 g

Fat: 3 g

Carbohydrate: 4 g

Fiber: 2 g

Excellent source: Vitamin A, Folic Acid

Good source: Iron

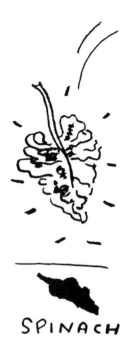

SPINACH

1. Flatten chicken slightly using fleshy side of your fist. Heat butter in a large nonstick frying pan set over medium-high heat. When butter is bubbly, add chicken and sauté until lightly golden, about 3 minutes per side. Remove chicken from pan. Stir in wine, bouillon cube, tarragon, Dijon and garlic. Reduce heat to medium and stir ingredients until blended. Boil gently, uncovered, for about 3 minutes.

2. Return chicken to pan. Cover and simmer until chicken feels springy, about 6 to 7 minutes, turning chicken halfway through. Remove chicken to a plate and cover to keep it warm. Boil sauce over medium-high heat, uncovered, until sauce is reduced to about ½ cup, for about 5 minutes. Meanwhile, clean spinach. Do not dry. When sauce is reduced, stir in sour cream if you like a creamy sauce and heat until hot. Do not boil. Taste and add more seasonings, if needed.

3. Pour sauce over chicken. Immediately add spinach to pan and stir often over medium-high heat until spinach is wilted and hot. Sprinkle with salt and pepper and serve alongside chicken.

FOCUS ON FOLATE

Folic acid (folate) is a key vitamin in lowering risk of birth defects, heart disease and cancer. These recipes are excellent sources of this vital vitamin.

Moroccan Chicken with Couscous

Couscous is actually a tiny pasta that contains only a trace of fat, and you don't have to cook it, just stir it into a hot liquid and let stand for 5 minutes. This easy-fix dinner is high in fiber and rich in folic acid.

PREPARATION TIME: 15 MINUTES / COOKING TIME: 30 MINUTES

MAKES: 4 SERVINGS

1 large onion, cut into thin wedges

4 crushed garlic cloves

1 tsp each of cinnamon, cumin and nutmeg

¼ tsp salt

6 chicken thighs, skin removed, or 4 skinless boneless chicken breasts

1 cup chicken bouillon or broth

1 cup orange juice

1 tbsp honey

3 carrots

1 cup uncooked couscous

4 green onions, thickly sliced

1. Place onion and garlic in a large nonstick frying pan. Sprinkle them with seasonings and place chicken on top. Add bouillon, orange juice and honey, then place pan over medium-high heat. Cook, uncovered, stirring onion occasionally, for 10 minutes, turning chicken halfway through. This will sweeten onion and reduce liquid slightly. Meanwhile, thinly slice carrots. Add carrots to pan as soon as they are sliced.

2. After onion has cooked for 10 minutes, partially cover pan and reduce heat to medium-low. Simmer, turning chicken partway through, until chicken feels springy, about 10 to 15 minutes. Remove chicken to a heated plate and cover with foil to keep warm. Stir couscous and green onions into pan juices, cover and turn off heat. Let stand for 5 minutes and fluff with a fork. Serve chicken on couscous.

FIERY FAJITA CHICKEN BAKE

Thinly slice 1 onion and 1 green pepper. Scatter them in a 9 x 13-inch (3-L) baking dish. Stir 7½-oz (213-mL) can tomato sauce with 1 cup salsa, 2 teaspoons chili powder, 2 teaspoons ground cumin, 1 teaspoon sugar, ½ teaspoon dried leaf oregano and ½ teaspoon salt. Pour over vegetables. Remove skin from 6 chicken breasts or legs. Arrange on top of tomato-vegetable mixture. Cover with foil. Bake in center of 400°F (200°C) oven for 30 minutes. Uncover and reduce heat to 350°F (180°C). Continue baking, basting often, until chicken is springy, about 35 to 45 more minutes. Place chicken on a serving plate. Stir sauce and spoon over top. *Serves 6.*

PER SERVING

Calories: 403

Protein: 29 g

Fat: 5 g

Carbohydrate: 59 g

Fiber: 5 g

Excellent source: Vitamin A, Folic Acid

Good source: Vitamin C, Iron

Easy Oven-Barbecued Chicken Dinner

Oven dinners serve up satisfying comfort with minimal fuss. A bottled barbecue sauce spruced up with beer and drizzled over chicken breasts, onions and sweet potatoes delivers old-fashioned barbecue flavor with less than an hour's baking time.

PREPARATION TIME: 15 MINUTES / ROASTING TIME: 45 MINUTES
MAKES: 4 SERVINGS

4 chicken breasts, bone-in
4 large cooking onions
4 sweet potatoes
Olive oil
Dried rosemary
½ cup bottled barbecue sauce
⅓ cup beer

1. Preheat oven to 375°F (190°C). Line a large broiler pan with foil and grease lightly. Place chicken breasts in pan, removing skin if you wish. Peel onions and slice in half. Put onions, cut-side down, in pan. Peel sweet potatoes and cut into halves or quarters, lengthwise, forming long wedges. Brush cut surfaces of potatoes with oil and sprinkle generously with rosemary. Add to pan.

2. Stir barbecue sauce with beer until evenly blended. Generously brush over chicken and onions, saving some sauce for basting. Bake, uncovered, in preheated oven for 45 to 55 minutes, brushing onions and chicken with remaining sauce at least every 15 minutes.

ESSENTIAL FAT

Fats are essential to keep our bodies functioning well. They are sources of essential fatty acids and aid in the absorption of the fat-soluble vitamins, A, D, E and K. Health professionals recommend we consume less than 30% of our calories from fat.

PER SERVING
WITHOUT SKIN

Calories: 348

Protein: 32 g

Fat: 2 g

Carbohydrate: 49 g

Fiber: 8 g

Excellent source: Vitamin A, Vitamin C

Good source: Folic Acid

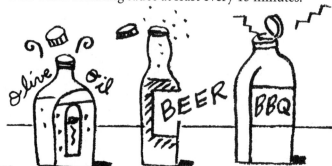

Terrific Teriyaki Chicken

Brimming with Oriental flavors, this is low-fat fare at its best.

PREPARATION TIME: 15 MINUTES / COOKING TIME: 20 MINUTES

MAKES: 4 SERVINGS

1 tsp sesame oil, preferably dark

4 skinless boneless chicken breasts

2 tbsp each of soy sauce and sherry

1 tsp granulated sugar

Pinch of ground ginger, or 1½ tsp finely
   chopped fresh ginger

1 small head broccoli

1 red pepper

3 green onions, thinly sliced

1. Heat oil in a large nonstick frying pan set over medium heat. Sauté chicken until golden, about 5 minutes per side. Add soy sauce, sherry, sugar and ginger. Cover and simmer over low heat for 5 minutes.

2. Meanwhile, cut broccoli into florets. Seed and thinly slice pepper. Add broccoli and pepper to simmering chicken. Cover and simmer for 5 more minutes or until vegetables are done as you like. Sprinkle with green onions. Great over rice.

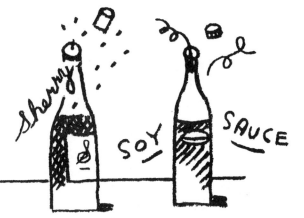

FAST ITALIAN CHICKEN

Pour 14 oz (398 mL) spaghetti sauce (about 2 cups) into a large wide saucepan. Set over medium heat. Place 4 large skinless chicken breasts, bone-side up, in pan. Cover and bring to a gentle boil. Stir in ¼ cup (125 g) sliced fresh mushrooms, 2 diced green peppers, ¼ teaspoon Italian seasoning and ¼ teaspoon hot red pepper flakes. Cover and simmer over low heat, turning chicken several times, until it is springy to the touch, about 25 to 35 minutes. Remove chicken to a platter and toss sauce with hot cooked pasta or spoon over rice. Sprinkle with Parmesan. *Serves 4.*

PER SERVING

Calories:	190
Protein:	31 g
Fat:	3 g
Carbohydrate:	9 g
Fiber:	3 g
Excellent source:	Vitamin C, Folic Acid
Good source:	Vitamin A

Spicy Pork and Peppers

For those nights when you crave something hot 'n' peppery, there's no need to stop for Mexican takeout. Start with a lean pork tenderloin and bell peppers and you can have a satisfying entrée on the table in less than 15 minutes. For a fast start, keep a pork tenderloin in the freezer, and defrost it in the microwave just until it can be easily sliced.

PREPARATION TIME: 10 MINUTES / COOKING TIME: 10 MINUTES
MAKES: 2 TO 3 SERVINGS

1 onion
2 tsp olive oil
1 pork tenderloin, about ¾ lb (375 g)
1 tsp each of minced fresh garlic and grated ginger, or 1½ tsp each of bottled minced garlic and ginger
¼ tsp hot red pepper flakes
½ tsp curry powder
½ cup dry white wine
2 small peppers, preferably 1 red and 1 green

1. Slice onion in half through the root. Place cut side down on cutting board and thinly slice. Heat oil in a large frying pan set over medium-low heat. Add onion, and cook, stirring occasionally. Meanwhile, slice tenderloin into ¼-inch rounds. Slice rounds into bite-size strips.

2. Add tenderloin to onion along with garlic, ginger, red pepper flakes and curry powder. Increase heat to medium. Stir frequently until pork is lightly browned, about 4 minutes. Add wine. Increase heat to medium-high. Slice peppers into strips and add them. Stir frequently until peppers are tender-crisp. Serve over steamed rice tossed with green peas or sliced green onions and a mango salad.

INSTANT FLAVOR BOOSTERS

Check supermarkets for bottles of minced garlic, chopped ginger, and a mixture of minced garlic and ginger.

Minced Garlic
• Add to hamburgers, meat loaves, spaghetti sauces and salad dressings.

• Add to butter or oil when sautéing chicken breasts or making a stir-fry.

• Rub over chicken skin, roasts or a rack of lamb before roasting.

Chopped Ginger
• Add to marinades, sauces for chicken or fish, and dressings for fruit or Oriental salads.

• Simmer in butter or olive oil, then sauté chicken, shrimp, or apple or pear wedges.

• Blend with sour cream or whipped cream cheese for fruit dips, or sauces for chicken or grilled fish.

PER SERVING

Calories:	204
Protein:	25 g
Fat:	6 g
Carbohydrate:	7 g
Fiber:	2 g
Excellent source:	Vitamin C

Fast Maple-Mustard Pork Chops and Squash Purée

Richly glazed pork chops with a bright purée of squash on the side are a cinch to make. Use maple syrup cut with mustard for the glaze, and enliven frozen puréed squash with orange zest and allspice.

PREPARATION TIME: 20 MINUTES / COOKING TIME: 25 MINUTES
MAKES: 2 TO 4 SERVINGS

4 thin pork chops, about ½-inch thick
2 to 3 tsp olive oil
¼ cup pure maple syrup
1 tsp dry mustard
Pinches of salt and freshly ground black pepper
12-oz (400-g) pkg frozen puréed cooked squash
1 to 2 tsp butter
Finely grated peel of 1 small orange
Pinches of nutmeg and allspice

1. Brown chops in oil in a frying pan set over medium-high heat, about 3 to 5 minutes per side. Reduce heat to medium and cook, uncovered, until done as you like, about 5 minutes per side. Remove chops to a platter. Drain fat from pan.

2. Add maple syrup and mustard to pan drippings. Whisk until blended. Return chops to pan and simmer until richly glazed, about 2 minutes per side. Add salt and pepper to taste.

3. While chops are cooking, cook squash according to package directions. Stir in butter, orange peel, and pinches of nutmeg, allspice, salt and pepper. Great with rice or baked potato.

MEXICAN-SPICED BEANS 'N' RICE

Chop 1 onion, 1 celery stalk and 1 red pepper. Sauté in 1 teaspoon olive oil with 1 crushed garlic clove for 3 minutes. Add entire contents of a 19-oz (540-mL) can kidney beans, ¼ teaspoon oregano and ¼ teaspoon chili powder. Stir gently until hot. Serve over rice. *Serves 4.*

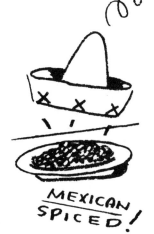

MEXICAN SPICED!

PER SERVING

Calories: 246	
Protein: 20 g	
Fat: 8 g	
Carbohydrate: 24 g	
Fiber: 2 g	
Excellent source: Vitamin A	

Grilled Dijon Flank Steak with Spuds and Peppers

To add real zing to this easy broiler recipe given to us by Chatelaine's editor, Rona Maynard, we jazzed up Dijon mustard with fresh ginger and a touch of soy, then slathered it on flank steak. Juicy flank steak is a good buy, and there's no fat to trim. Our delicious coating adds only zesty taste.

PREPARATION TIME: 15 MINUTES / MARINATING TIME: OVERNIGHT

MICROWAVING TIME: 6 MINUTES / BROILING TIME: 16 MINUTES

MAKES: 4 TO 6 SERVINGS

3 tbsp Dijon mustard

1 tbsp soy sauce

1 tbsp grated fresh ginger, or 1 tsp ground ginger

½ tsp dried leaf thyme

2-lb (1-kg) flank steak

½ tsp coarsely ground black pepper

4 small baking potatoes

2 small peppers, preferably red

1 tbsp olive oil

Pinches of salt and cayenne pepper

1. Stir Dijon with soy sauce, ginger and thyme. Spread mixture over both sides of steak, then sprinkle it with black pepper. For maximum flavor penetration, put steak, folding in half if needed, in a resealable plastic bag or in a flat dish. Seal bag or cover dish with plastic wrap. Refrigerate for several hours or overnight.

2. When ready to cook, preheat broiler. Place whole unpeeled potatoes in microwave and cook on high for 6 to 8 minutes or until almost soft. Wrap in a tea towel and let sit 2 minutes. Slice into thirds, lengthwise. Place in a bowl. Seed peppers, cut into thirds and add to potatoes. Drizzle with oil. Grind lots of black pepper over top. Sprinkle with salt and cayenne. Toss until evenly coated.

FOUR-PEPPER STEAK

Heat 1 to 2 tablespoons olive oil in a large frying pan. Press ½ teaspoon freshly ground black pepper into both sides of 4 cubed or quick-fry steaks. Cook over medium-high heat 2 minutes per side. Remove steaks and cover to keep warm. Add ¾ cup Beaujolais, ⅛ teaspoon cayenne pepper and a generous pinch of salt to pan. Boil, uncovered, until wine is reduced to ¼ cup, about 3 minutes. Stir in ½ cup julienne strips red pepper and ½ cup julienne strips green pepper. Pour over steaks and serve. *Serves 2 to 4.*

PER SERVING

Calories: 382	
Protein: 38 g	
Fat: 15 g	
Carbohydrate: 24 g	
Fiber: 2 g	
Excellent source: Vitamin C, Iron	

3. Place steak, covered with marinade coating, on broiler tray. Broil on top rack until seared, about 8 minutes per side for medium-rare. Flank steak cooked more than medium tends to be tough.

4. Spread potatoes and peppers out on a broiler pan. Broil along with steak until golden, about 4 to 5 minutes per side. Place steak on a cutting board and thinly slice meat across the grain. Serve right away.

New-Style Easy Stuffed Peppers

A zesty veggie-packed hit, especially in fall when peppers are cheap and plentiful.

PREPARATION TIME: 20 MINUTES / COOKING TIME: 6 MINUTES
BAKING TIME: 35 MINUTES / MAKES: 3 SERVINGS

½ lb (250 g) ground chicken or turkey

1 tsp ground cumin

¼ tsp salt

¼ tsp hot red pepper flakes (optional)

3 medium-size peppers, preferably different colors

19-oz (540-mL) can tomatoes

¾ cup uncooked, instant or quick-cooking rice

½ cup kernel corn, frozen or canned

2 green onions, sliced

1. Preheat oven to 375°F (190°C). Crumble chicken into a large nonstick frying pan set over medium heat. Sprinkle chicken with seasonings. Cook, working with a fork to keep chicken crumbly, until it loses its pink color, about 6 to 8 minutes.

2. Meanwhile, slice peppers in half, lengthwise through stem. Remove stems and seeds. Drain liquid from tomatoes into a measuring cup. Add water to tomato juice to bring it up to the ¾-cup level.

3. Put tomatoes in a large mixing bowl. Break them up, using a fork. Add tomato liquid to bowl. Stir in cooked chicken, uncooked rice, corn and green onions.

EGGPLANT STEAKS FOR TWO

Slice 1 large unpeeled eggplant lengthwise into ½-inch slices. Sprinkle each side with a pinch of salt. Arrange slices in an ungreased 9 x 13-inch (3-L) baking dish. Sprinkle with ½ teaspoon each of dried basil, leaf oregano, sugar and garlic powder. Top with 2 or 3 thickly sliced large tomatoes. Sprinkle with 1 cup crumbled feta or chèvre. Bake, uncovered, in bottom of 375°F (190°C) oven until eggplant is tender when pierced with a fork, about 30 to 35 minutes. *Serves 2.*

PER SERVING

Calories: 396

Protein: 21 g

Fat: 9 g

Carbohydrate: 59 g

Fiber: 6 g

Excellent source: Vitamin A, Vitamin C

Good source: Folic Acid, Iron

4. Spoon mixture into pepper halves, mounding it in center of each pepper half. Arrange filled pepper halves in an ungreased 9 x 13-inch (3-L) baking dish. Cover with a tent of foil and bake in center of oven until peppers are tender when pierced with a fork, about 35 to 40 minutes.

FOR VEGETARIANS: *Omit the chicken and stir in more corn and some grated cheese.*

EXPRESS GRAINS

Fast-fixing grains — from 5-minute couscous to packaged rolls of polenta — are adding healthy textures to everyday dinners. Thanks to new quick-cooking wild rice, bulgur, couscous and quinoa (keen-wa) being sold in many supermarkets, it's faster to do a toss or salad with one of these nutrient-rich grains than to cook pasta. Here are some quick ways to add zesty taste to fashionable side dishes.

TABBOULEH

Stir 2 cups cooked quinoa or bulgur with 2 finely chopped tomatoes and 1 cup chopped parsley. Stir in a mixture of 2 tablespoons lemon juice, 1 tablespoon olive oil, 1 crushed garlic clove and pinches of salt and black pepper. *Makes 3 cups.*

CHEESY POLENTA

Slice a 1-lb (500-g) polenta roll into ½-inch slices. Dip each into freshly grated Parmesan or Romano cheese. Heat 1 tablespoon olive oil with 1 crushed garlic clove in a nonstick frying pan set over medium heat. Sauté slices until golden. *Makes 9 slices.*

MEXICAN BREAKFAST

Coarsely chop a 1-lb (500-g) polenta roll and place in a saucepan with ⅔ cup water, ¼ teaspoon ground cumin and a pinch of hot red pepper flakes. Cook over medium heat, stirring frequently until smooth and hot. Stir in ½ cup grated old cheddar cheese and 2 tablespoons chopped fresh coriander. Serve topped with 4 poached or fried eggs and drizzled with warm tomato salsa. *Makes 4 servings.*

QUINOA PILAF

Sauté 1 small chopped onion, ¼ cup pine nuts or slivered almonds, and 1 crushed garlic clove in 1 tablespoon olive oil in a frying pan set over medium heat. When onion is soft, stir in 2 cups hot cooked quinoa, ¼ teaspoon salt and a pinch of cayenne. *Makes 3½ cups.*

CONFETTI WILD RICE

Sauté 1 chopped small red pepper and 1 chopped small yellow pepper in 1 tablespoon butter in a frying pan set over medium heat. When peppers are cooked but still firm, stir in 2 cups hot cooked wild rice, 2 thinly sliced green onions and ¼ tsp salt. *Makes 3 cups.*

FRUITED COUSCOUS

Bring 1½ cups chicken bouillon, ½ cup chopped dried apricots and ¼ teaspoon grated orange peel to a boil in a small saucepan. Stir in 1 cup dry couscous. Cover, remove from heat and let stand for 5 minutes. Fluff with a fork and stir in 2 tablespoons currants or raisins. *Makes 3⅓ cups.*

Couscous with Stir-Fried Spring Vegetables

A very fast vegetarian meal for two from Calgary chef Ken Canavan.

PREPARATION TIME: 10 MINUTES / COOKING TIME: 7 MINUTES
MAKES: 2 SERVINGS

1¼ cups water
¼ tsp salt
1 cup couscous
¼ cup currants (optional)
2 tsp olive oil
2 large crushed garlic cloves
3 cups sliced mixed vegetables, such as broccoli, peppers, celery and zucchini
½ tsp paprika
Pinch of cayenne pepper
2 tbsp freshly squeezed lemon juice
2 green onions, thinly sliced

1. Bring water and salt to a boil in a saucepan set over medium-high heat, or boil water and salt in a large bowl in the microwave. Remove pan from heat. Stir in couscous and currants. Cover and set aside for at least 5 minutes.

2. Heat oil in a wide nonstick frying pan set over medium heat. Add garlic and vegetables. Stir-fry until done as you like, about 2 minutes. Sprinkle vegetables with paprika and cayenne and stir until they are evenly distributed. Remove from heat. Stir lemon juice and green onions into couscous. Serve sautéed vegetables on a bed of couscous.

GREAT GRAINS

Bulgur is wheat kernels that have been steamed, dried and crushed. It has a nutty taste and firm texture when cooked for 5 minutes.

Polenta, or cornmeal "mush," is a mainstay of the Italian diet. Cooked with water or stock and salt into a thick porridge, it's great flavored with Parmesan, herbs and crushed chilies. Now sold in many grocery stores in a 1-lb (500-g) roll, it can simply be sliced and quickly sautéed in olive oil or butter until golden.

Quinoa is higher in protein than most grains and cooks in 10 minutes. The tiny grains have a caviar-like texture.

PER SERVING

Calories:	435
Protein:	14 g
Fat:	5 g
Carbohydrate:	83 g
Fiber:	8 g
Excellent source:	Vitamin C, Folic Acid
Good source:	Iron

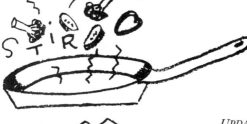

Vegetarian Mushroom and Red Pepper Cabbage Rolls

No apologies needed for the lack of meat in these healthy cabbage rolls. Nippy cheddar rounds out the mushroom flavor and adds essential protein. One batch of these rolls makes enough to feed a hungry crowd or for several freezer meals.

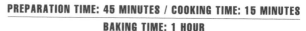

PREPARATION TIME: 45 MINUTES / COOKING TIME: 15 MINUTES

BAKING TIME: 1 HOUR

MAKES: 24 CABBAGE ROLLS, ABOUT 12 SERVINGS

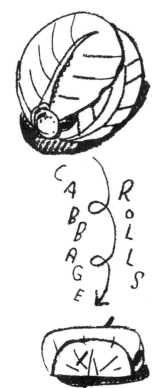

1 onion

½ lb (250 g) mushrooms

2 large carrots

1 red pepper, seeded

1½ tsp olive oil

2 crushed garlic cloves

½ tsp salt

¼ to ½ tsp hot red pepper flakes

10-oz (284-g) bag or 1 to 2 bunches fresh spinach, about 7 cups loosely packed leaves

2 cups cooked rice

4 cups grated old cheddar, fontina or mixture of cheeses, such as mozzarella and cheddar

1 medium head cabbage

3 cups thick spaghetti sauce, or a 24-oz (750-mL) jar

½ tsp each of dried leaf basil and leaf oregano

PER SERVING (2 ROLLS)

Calories: 297

Protein: 14 g

Fat: 15 g

Carbohydrate: 28 g

Fiber: 4 g

Excellent source: Vitamin A, Vitamin C, Folic Acid, Calcium

Good source: Iron

1. Coarsely chop onion and set aside. Chop mushrooms, carrots and pepper. Heat oil in a large wide heavy-bottomed saucepan set over medium heat. Add onion and garlic and sauté until softened, about 5 minutes. Add chopped vegetables, salt and red pepper flakes. Sauté, uncovered, stirring often, until most of moisture on bottom of pan has evaporated, about 8 to 10 minutes.

2. Meanwhile, remove any stems from spinach and discard. Wash leaves thoroughly, drain and coarsely chop. Chopped spinach should measure about 4 cups. Add spinach to vegetables and stir frequently just until spinach is wilted, about 2 minutes. Remove mixture from heat and add rice. Sprinkle with 2 cups grated cheese and stir gently until evenly mixed. Set aside to cool slightly while continuing with recipe.

3. Preheat oven to 350°F (180°C). Prepare cabbage leaves using one of the methods given below. Cut out hard center ribs at bottom of larger wilted cabbage leaves. Small leaves can be overlapped to be large enough for rolling. Place 2 to 4 tablespoons filling in center of each leaf, depending on its size. Tuck sides in and roll up. Place rolls close together, seam-side down, in a 9 x 13-inch (3-L) baking dish.

4. Stir spaghetti sauce with basil and oregano and spoon over rolls. Cover loosely with foil. Bake in center of oven for 30 minutes. Then, uncover and sprinkle with remaining 2 cups grated cheese. Bake, uncovered, until sauce is bubbly and cheese is golden, about 30 more minutes.

CABBAGE ROLLS MADE EASY

Cabbage leaves must be partially cooked or wilted in order to wrap around filling. Here are 3 methods.

STOVE-TOP

Half fill a large saucepan with water and bring to a boil over high heat. Do not remove core from cabbage. Deeply embed a long cooking fork into core to provide a handle for dipping cabbage. Submerge cabbage in boiling water. After 2 to 3 minutes, remove cabbage and hold under cold running water. When cool enough to touch, carefully remove wilted leaves and drain. Repeat plunging, cooling and removing until all the leaves are wilted.

MICROWAVE

Place whole cabbage on a microwave-safe dish and microwave, uncovered, on high for 3 to 5 minutes or until outer leaves are bright green and partially cooked. Remove cabbage and hold under cold running water. When cool enough to touch, carefully remove wilted leaves and drain. Repeat microwaving, cooling and removing leaves until all are wilted.

FREEZER

Place whole cabbage, uncovered, in the freezer. Leave overnight. Defrost at room temperature. Leaves can easily be rolled. We find leaves wilted using this method occasionally have a strong taste.

Lusty Vegetable Stew with Feta and Basil

Mediterranean cuisine is in the spotlight, partly because it's based on vegetables and straightforward flavors. This hearty stew is substantial enough to star in a fast supper. Garlic bread is all you need on the side. Wind up with a tart lemon sherbet.

PREPARATION TIME: 15 MINUTES / COOKING TIME: 30 MINUTES

MAKES: 4 SERVINGS

1 to 2 tbsp olive oil
2 crushed garlic cloves
1 onion, coarsely chopped
2 peppers, cored and chopped
2 carrots, sliced
2 potatoes, peeled and thinly sliced
3 thin zucchini, cut into 1-inch pieces
28-oz (796-mL) can plum tomatoes, including juice
1 tsp each of leaf thyme and granulated sugar
Generous grinding of black pepper
½ to 1 cup crumbled feta cheese
¼ cup chopped fresh basil (optional)

1. In a large wide saucepan, heat 1 tablespoon oil over medium heat. Add garlic, onion, peppers and carrots. Sauté for 5 minutes, stirring often, adding more oil only if needed. Stir in remaining ingredients, except cheese and basil. Bring mixture to a boil.

2. Cover, reduce heat and simmer gently, until vegetables are done as you like, about 20 minutes. Stir occasionally. Serve in soup bowls sprinkled with cheese and basil.

CRUSTY GARLIC BREAD

Preheat oven to 400°F (200°C). In a small bowl, stir 2 tablespoons olive oil or butter with ½ teaspoon garlic powder and a generous grinding of black pepper. Cut 1 small crusty baguette into thick slices but do not cut all the way through to the bottom. Spread cut surfaces with mixture. Wrap in foil. Bake for 5 to 10 minutes or until heated through.

PER SERVING

Calories: 277

Protein: 10 g

Fat: 11 g

Carbohydrate: 39 g

Fiber: 7 g

Excellent source: Vitamin A, Vitamin C, Folic Acid

Good source: Calcium, Iron

Entertaining Made Easy

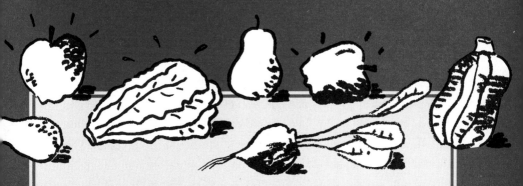

Incredible Classy Curried Shrimp

Low-Fat Jazzy Jambalaya

Lime-Ginger Chicken with Spicy Mango Sauce

Beaujolais Steak and Oven Frites for Two

Classy Coriander Chicken Curry

Phyllo Vegetable Pie

Philip's Upscale Gumbo

Roast Turkey à Deux

Rosé Pork Roast with Fall Vegetables

Incredible Classy Curried Shrimp

What's so amazing about this curry? The few ingredients needed and the speed with which you can create a very impressive party dish. Perfect as a small first course or the entire entrée — no side dishes needed. And you can make it completely ahead of a dinner party, adding the shrimp when you reheat.

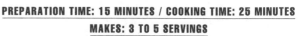

PREPARATION TIME: 15 MINUTES / COOKING TIME: 25 MINUTES
MAKES: 3 TO 5 SERVINGS

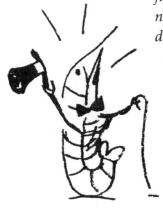

14-oz (398-mL) can light coconut milk

2 to 3 tsp curry paste, or 1 tsp each of curry powder and cumin

1 large onion

6 plum tomatoes, or 3 regular tomatoes, or 28-oz (796-mL) can plum tomatoes

2 peppers, preferably yellow

1 lb (500 g) fresh tiger shrimp or frozen medium-size shrimp

1 bunch fresh spinach, 4 cups coarsely shredded

6 thin green onions

2 limes

1 lb (400 g) pasta, cooked, or 3 cups cooked rice (optional)

Chopped fresh coriander (optional)

PER SERVING
WITH PASTA

Calories: 480

Protein: 27 g

Fat: 7 g

Carbohydrate: 77 g

Fiber: 7 g

Excellent source: Vitamin A, Vitamin C, Folic Acid, Iron

PER SERVING
WITHOUT PASTA

Calories: 184

Protein: 17 g

Fat: 6 g

Carbohydrate: 18 g

Fiber: 4 g

Excellent source: Vitamin A, Vitamin C, Folic Acid, Iron

1. Pour coconut milk into a large wide saucepan. Set over medium-high heat. Stir in 2 teaspoons of curry paste or curry powder and cumin. To thicken sauce, boil gently, uncovered and stirring occasionally, while preparing the vegetables. (Curry paste comes in many different strengths. Start with 2 teaspoons as we suggested, then after sauce has cooked 5 minutes, taste and stir in more paste, if you like. We've used from 2 teaspoons to 2 tablespoons. Remember the flavor will be greatly decreased when mixed with pasta.)

2. Peel and coarsely chop onion and immediately stir into boiling sauce. Slice fresh tomatoes in half and squeeze them over the sink to discard all juice and seeds. Coarsely chop tomatoes, then stir into boiling sauce. Or drain can of tomatoes well. While tomatoes are still in the can, cut them into 2 or 3 pieces each. Gently press them with a fork and drain again. Add to boiling sauce. Slice peppers into thin bite-size strips and stir in. Let the mixture continue boiling gently, uncovered and stirring often, until thick enough to lightly coat pasta.

3. Meanwhile, shell fresh shrimp or place frozen shrimp in a sieve and rinse with warm water until ice crystals disappear. Coarsely shred spinach leaves. They should measure about 4 cups. If green onions are large, slice in half lengthwise, then slice into 1-inch pieces. Slice 1 lime in half and the other into wedges.

4. When sauce is thick and about 5 minutes before serving, stir shrimp into boiling sauce. Continue stirring gently and often over medium-high heat just until most of the shrimp have become bright pink. This should take no more than 3 minutes. Immediately remove from the heat. (Shrimp will continue cooking.) Add all the spinach and green onions. If serving with pasta, stir in the hot pasta. Turn onto a large platter or individual plates. If using rice, pour over hot rice on a platter. Squeeze juice from 1 lime over top. Scatter coriander over top and serve immediately.

MAKE AHEAD: *Complete Step 2, cooking sauce until thick enough to coat pasta. Remove from heat, cover and leave at room temperature for several hours or refrigerate up to 2 days. Reheat over low heat. Proceed with recipe.*

CHICKEN, TOO: *If using as an entrée, chicken is a great addition. Slice 2 skinless boneless chicken breasts into thin strips. At the point of the recipe where you would add shrimp, stir in chicken instead. Stir often for 4 minutes. Then, add shrimp and proceed with recipe.*

LIGHT COCONUT MILK

Wonderfully flavorful coconut milk is used in many Asian cuisines to add a seductive creaminess to a dish. Grated fresh coconut is pressed and the thick extract from the first pressing is called coconut cream. Subsequent thinner pressings are called coconut milk. High in saturated fat, coconut milk is now available in a light version containing 40% less fat and calories than regular coconut milk. Coconut milk is sold in Asian or West Indian stores, as well as in many supermarkets. Check the label so you don't confuse unsweetened *coconut cream* with the heavily sweetened *cream of coconut* that is used for piña coladas and desserts.

Low-Fat Jazzy Jambalaya

Try low-fat smoked turkey instead of bacon to give a classic smoky taste to this big-batch party jambalaya.

PREPARATION TIME: 25 MINUTES / COOKING TIME: 45 MINUTES

MAKES: 14 CUPS (WITHOUT TURKEY OR SHRIMP)

1 tbsp olive oil

4 skinless boneless chicken breasts

2 large red or white onions, chopped

4 large crushed garlic cloves, or 2 tbsp bottled minced garlic

6 ripe tomatoes, about 4 cups chopped, or 2 (28-oz/796-mL) cans tomatoes, drained

4 green peppers, seeded

4 celery stalks

3 cups chicken broth or bouillon

2 cups uncooked long-grain rice

1 tbsp ground cumin

1½ tsp salt

1 tsp each of dried leaf oregano, leaf thyme and hot pepper sauce

½ lb (250 g) smoked turkey or chicken, cut into ½-inch cubes (optional)

1 lb (500 g) fresh or frozen shelled shrimp (optional)

1. Pour oil into a large wide saucepan. Sauté chicken breasts until golden, about 5 minutes per side. Remove chicken from pan and add onions and garlic to pan. Sauté, stirring often, until onions are softened.

2. Meanwhile, coarsely chop fresh unpeeled tomatoes and peppers. Slice celery into ½-inch pieces. Stir half of celery and peppers and all of fresh or drained canned tomatoes into onions. Break up canned tomatoes. Cook, stirring often to prevent burning. Slice chicken into bite-size pieces and stir into simmering sauce. Stir in broth, rice, cumin, salt, oregano, thyme and hot pepper sauce.

TOMATO 'N' CHEDDAR FOCACCIA SQUARES

Place a ¾-lb (400-g) focaccia bread or a pizza shell on a baking sheet. Spread with ½ cup spaghetti sauce or arrange 2 large, thinly sliced tomatoes on top, overlapping slightly. Sprinkle with 1 teaspoon Italian seasoning, ¼ teaspoon hot red pepper flakes, then ½ cup grated old cheddar cheese. Bake on bottom rack of preheated 375°F (190°C) oven until golden, about 20 minutes. Serve immediately. *Makes 12 squares.*

PER CUP

Calories: 196	
Protein: 13 g	
Fat: 2 g	
Carbohydrate: 31 g	
Fiber: 3 g	
Excellent source: Vitamin C	

3. Cover and bring to a boil. Reduce heat to medium-low and simmer for 15 minutes. Stir in remaining celery, peppers and smoked turkey. Continue cooking, covered, for 10 more minutes or until most of liquid has evaporated. If serving right away, stir in shrimp and continue cooking until shrimp are bright pink, about 5 minutes. If storing in the refrigerator or freezing, do not add shrimp until casserole is reheated. You can refrigerate for up to 2 days. If jambalaya is frozen, however, defrost it in the refrigerator. This may take 2 days for all ice crystals to melt. Then, place cold jambalaya in 2 casserole dishes, each holding about 8 cups. Cover and place in a preheated 325°F (160°C) oven for 1¼ hours. Stir every 15 minutes. Stir in shrimp and continue heating until shrimp are bright pink, about 7 minutes. To freshen taste, stir in a little crushed garlic and chopped fresh herbs, if needed. For texture, stir in finely chopped fresh peppers or celery.

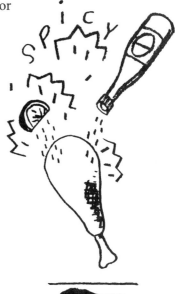

Lime-Ginger Chicken with Spicy Mango Sauce

Treat chicken to a blender lime, ginger and rum marinade that smacks of the Tropics.

PREPARATION TIME: 15 MINUTES / MARINATING TIME: 1 HOUR
BAKING TIME: 45 MINUTES / MAKES: 4 SERVINGS

4 chicken breasts or legs

MARINADE
2 limes
1 onion, quartered
1 large garlic clove
1-inch piece fresh ginger, or ½ tsp ground ginger
2 tbsp each of rum, brown sugar and soy sauce
1 tbsp olive oil
1 tsp hot chili-garlic sauce or hot pepper sauce
¼ tsp each of allspice, cinnamon, nutmeg and salt
¼ cup chopped fresh coriander

PER SERVING
(WITHOUT SKIN)

Calories: 169

Protein: 27 g

Fat: 3 g

Carbohydrate: 6 g

Fiber: trace

SPICY MANGO SAUCE
1 lime
1 tbsp brown sugar
¼ to ½ tsp hot pepper sauce
2 ripe mangoes, peeled and chopped
½ cup chopped fresh coriander
2 green onions, thinly sliced

1. Remove skin from chicken, if you wish. Using a sharp knife, slash chicken 3 or 4 times, crosswise, through to a depth of about ½ inch, forming cuts about 1 inch apart. Place chicken in a dish or resealable plastic bag.

2. Squeeze juice from 2 limes. In a food processor or blender, combine lime juice with remaining marinade ingredients. Whirl until very finely chopped. Measure out ¼ cup, cover it and set it aside in refrigerator. Pour remaining marinade over chicken and turn pieces until they are evenly coated. Cover dish or seal bag. Refrigerate for at least 1 hour or up to 1 day. Turn chicken or bag at least once during marinating time.

3. Meanwhile, to prepare Spicy Mango Sauce, squeeze juice from 1 lime. Stir with sugar and hot pepper sauce until sugar is dissolved. Then stir in mangoes and coriander. Let sauce stand at room temperature while chicken is roasting. If making ahead, marinade can be left at room temperature for 2 to 3 hours or refrigerated up to a day.

4. Preheat oven to 375°F (190°C). For easy cleanup, use foil to line a broiling pan or a baking sheet with shallow sides. Place a rack on pan. Remove chicken from marinade, saving marinade, and place, bone-side down, on rack. Bake, uncovered, in center of oven for 15 minutes. Baste with reserved marinade, then continue baking until chicken is cooked as you like, about 30 to 35 more minutes. Stir green onions into Spicy Mango Sauce and serve sauce with chicken.

FIDDLEHEADS

In spring it's fun to search out these delicate, tightly coiled fern fronds. They make a wonderful feast and extras freeze well. Fiddleheads have a taste somewhere between asparagus and green beans. Wash well, then briefly steam or sauté until barely tender. Add a dab of butter or a squirt of lemon juice and a sprinkle of Parmesan cheese for best flavor. A good source of vitamins A and C.

Beaujolais Steak and Oven Frites for Two

Steak and pommes frites spell special dining in any language. Even novice cooks can produce a perfectly cooked steak with wine sauce and crisp chunky potatoes by following our surefire skillet method for the steaks while the potatoes crisp in the oven.

PREPARATION TIME: 15 MINUTES / BAKING TIME: 30 MINUTES
COOKING TIME: 13 MINUTES / MAKES: 2 SERVINGS

2 large baking potatoes
1 tbsp olive oil
Salt and freshly ground black pepper
2 tsp butter or olive oil
2 strip-loin or rib-eye steaks, at least 1 inch thick
½ cup Beaujolais or cabernet sauvignon
2 tbsp salsa, mild to hot, as you prefer

1. Adjust oven rack to lowest level. Preheat oven to 450°F (230°C). Scrub potatoes. Peel them only if you wish. Slice potatoes into ½-inch rounds, then into ½-inch strips. Pat dry and place in a bowl. Drizzle with oil and sprinkle generously with salt and pepper. Stir until evenly coated. Spread them on a baking sheet, preferably dark in color to speed browning. Bake on bottom rack of oven, turning 2 or 3 times, until browned and tender, about 30 to 35 minutes.

2. About 10 minutes before potatoes are cooked, set a heavy-bottomed frying pan over medium heat. When hot, put in butter and tilt pan to coat bottom. When butter bubbles, add steaks (cold from refrigerator) and fry until well browned, about 3 minutes per side for rare or 5 minutes for medium steaks. Remove to heated plates. Pour wine into pan juices and increase heat to medium-high. Scrape all brown bits from bottom of pan. Stir in salsa and boil gently, stirring often, until mixture is thick enough to coat steaks, about 2 to 3 minutes. Pour over steaks and serve right away with oven frites.

NO GREEN, PLEASE

When potatoes are exposed to light or to warm temperatures, a substance called solanine turns them green. Don't eat the green part; it tastes bitter and eating large quantities can make you sick. Prevent potatoes from greening by storing them in a cool dark place.

GRILLED CHÈVRE TOMATOES

Slice ripe tomatoes in half and squeeze out seeds and juice. Place them on a baking sheet. Crumble a little chèvre over top and sprinkle with chopped fresh basil, oregano or chives. Grill under preheated broiler until cheese is golden, about 5 minutes. Beautiful with roast chicken, beef or steak.

PER SERVING

Calories: 546	
Protein: 33 g	
Fat: 24 g	
Carbohydrate: 41 g	
Fiber: 4 g	
Excellent source: Iron	
Good source: Vitamin C	

Classy Coriander Chicken Curry

No matter what the affair, this fabulous curry, which begins with roasting three aromatic seeds, will be the talk of the dinner.

PREPARATION TIME: 30 MINUTES / COOKING TIME: 55 MINUTES

MAKES: 6 SERVINGS

2 tsp each coriander seeds and cumin seeds

1 tsp each mustard seeds and black peppercorns

4 large chicken breasts, or 6 pieces of chicken

2 tsp olive oil

1 onion, coarsely chopped

1 jalapeño pepper, seeded and finely chopped (optional)

2 tbsp finely chopped ginger

4 crushed garlic cloves

14-oz (398-mL) can light or regular coconut milk

2 large tomatoes, seeded and chopped

1 tbsp freshly squeezed lime or lemon juice

1 tsp salt

½ tsp turmeric

¼ tsp cayenne pepper

3-inch cinnamon stick

2 apples, peeled and chopped

1 large red pepper

1 banana (optional)

½ cup light sour cream (optional)

½ to 1 cup chopped fresh coriander

1. Combine coriander seeds with cumin seeds, mustard seeds and peppercorns in a large wide heavy-bottomed frying pan. Do not add any liquid or fat. Place over medium heat and stir often until very fragrant, about 10 minutes. Grind seeds and peppercorns in a blender, mini chopper or peppermill. Set aside.

VITAMIN C CHOICES

Most of us rely on an orange or glass of orange juice for our daily fix of vitamin C. But, the following contain at least as much vitamin C as 1 orange: 1 cup cauliflower, broccoli or brussels sprouts, ½ cantaloupe, ½ papaya, 1 green pepper (red peppers have twice as much as green) or 1 cup strawberries.

PER SERVING

Calories: 209

Protein: 20 g

Fat: 7 g

Carbohydrate: 18 g

Fiber: 3 g

Excellent source: Vitamin C

Good source: Vitamin A

2. Meanwhile, remove fat and skin from chicken. Pour oil into pan that was used for dry roasting spices. Place pan over medium heat. When oil is hot, add chicken and sauté until golden-tinged, about 5 minutes per side. Then, add onion, jalapeño pepper, ginger and garlic. Sauté, stirring often, until onion is soft, about 5 minutes. Lower heat, if necessary, so garlic and ginger do not brown.

3. Add coconut milk, tomatoes, lime juice, seasonings, ground roasted spices and whole cinnamon stick. Cover and bring to a boil. Meanwhile, peel and chop apples. Immediately stir apples into sauce. Cover and reduce heat to low. Simmer, turning chicken once, until done as you like, about 30 to 40 minutes.

4. While chicken is simmering, seed pepper. Slice into thin strips, then cut into bite-size lengths. Slice banana into ¼-inch rounds. When chicken is done, remove to a bowl. Stir pepper strips into sauce. To thicken sauce, increase heat to medium-low. Boil gently, uncovered and stirring often. Remove chicken from bones and cut meat into bite-size pieces. When sauce is as thick as you like, remove cinnamon stick and stir in chicken and banana, if using. Stir in sour cream, if using, until blended. Stir in about half of fresh coriander. Serve over rice and sprinkle generously with remaining fresh coriander.

MAKE AHEAD: *Prepare sauce and stir in bite-size pieces of chicken. Refrigerate for up to 1 day. It can be frozen but texture of sauce will probably suffer a little. Add banana, sour cream and coriander after reheating.*

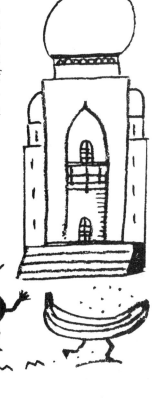

Phyllo Vegetable Pie

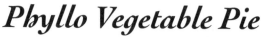

You won't miss the meat in this vegetarian dish. Flaky layers of phyllo surround layers of creamy rice and spinach, subtly spiced with the tastes of Morocco — cinnamon, raisins and lemon. This pie is a snap to make, even if you've never worked with phyllo before.

PREPARATION TIME: 30 MINUTES / COOKING TIME: 8 MINUTES
BAKING TIME: 1¼ HOURS / MAKES: 8 TO 12 WEDGES

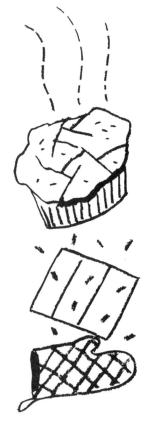

RICE LAYER
1 lemon
1 egg
2 cups cooked rice, about 1 cup dry rice, cooked
1 cup ricotta cheese, about ½ (1-lb/475-g) container
1 cup grated mozzarella cheese

SPINACH LAYER
1 tbsp olive oil or butter
2 onions, chopped
4 crushed garlic cloves
½ to 1 tsp hot red pepper flakes (optional)
2 (10-oz/284-g) pkgs fresh spinach leaves
½ cup raisins
½ tsp cinnamon
Pinch of salt
½ cup grated mozzarella cheese

ASSEMBLY
6 sheets phyllo pastry
4 to 6 tbsp olive oil or melted butter
1½ cups thick spaghetti sauce

PER WEDGE

Calories: 284	
Protein: 10 g	
Fat: 14 g	
Carbohydrate: 32 g	
Fiber: 3 g	
Excellent source: Vitamin A, Folic Acid	
Good source: Calcium, Iron	

1. To prepare rice layer, finely grate 1 teaspoon of peel from lemon and squeeze out 1 tablespoon juice. Beat egg in a mixing bowl and stir in cooked rice, ricotta, 1 cup grated mozzarella, lemon peel and juice.

2. To prepare spinach layer, heat oil in a large frying pan set over medium heat. Add onions, garlic and red pepper flakes. Sauté until onions have softened, about 5 minutes. Wash spinach and tear into bite-size pieces, discarding stems. Add spinach to softened onions and sprinkle with raisins, cinnamon and salt. Continue cooking, stirring occasionally, just until spinach is wilted, about 3 minutes. Remove from heat. Sir in ½ cup mozzarella.

3. Preheat oven to 375°F (190°C). To assemble pie, have fillings ready since phyllo dries out quickly. Lay 1 piece phyllo on a cutting board, covering remaining phyllo with plastic wrap until ready to use. Lightly brush both sides of phyllo sheet with oil. Place in a 9-inch (23-cm) oiled pie plate so one edge of phyllo is even with edge of plate, covering bottom and sides, and extending beyond the rim on the other side. Repeat with remaining phyllo, placing each sheet into pie plate so the longer ends are evenly spaced in a circular pattern around rim.

4. Pour half of rice mixture into bottom and gently smooth the top. Spread with half of the spinach mixture, then with ¾ cup spaghetti sauce. Repeat layers, ending with ¾ cup spaghetti sauce. Bring hanging ends of phyllo up and gently fold them over filling. Phyllo should have a rough appearance. Do not pat down edges of phyllo. Bake in center of oven until phyllo is golden and center of filling is hot, about 1¼ hours. Cool for 5 minutes before slicing into wedges. Since phyllo quickly loses its crispness, this pie is best served on the day it is baked.

MAKE AHEAD: *Pie can be prepared, then covered with plastic wrap or a tent of foil and refrigerated for up to 1 day. To bake, preheat oven to 375°F (190°C). Remove wrapping and bake cold pie in center of oven until center of filling is hot, about 1½ to 1¾ hours.*

SWISS CHARD

Related to beets, with a spinach-like appearance, chard's large leaves and sturdy stalk are succulent eating, especially when picked young. Wash thoroughly to remove any sand, briefly sauté with a bit of olive oil and garlic, then sprinkle with vinegar or lemon juice and a little brown sugar. A half cup of boiled Swiss chard contains generous amounts of beta-carotene and vitamin C, as well as iron, calcium and several other nutrients — all for only 18 calories and less than a gram of fat.

Philip's Upscale Gumbo

Our friend Philip Greey serves a mean gumbo — one of the best we've ever had. Adapted from the charming Sunshine Café in Captiva, Florida, Philip's creation can be made a day ahead if you want. Reheat when guests arrive. Add fish and seafood just before serving for that seductive fresh seafood taste.

PREPARATION TIME: 30 MINUTES / COOKING TIME: 55 MINUTES

MAKES: 4 TO 8 SERVINGS

2 tbsp olive oil

6 garlic cloves, minced or crushed

2 tbsp all-purpose flour

10-oz (284-mL) can chicken broth, or 2½ cups chicken bouillon

10-oz (284-mL) bottle clam juice

1 tsp dried leaf oregano

½ tsp each of dried basil, paprika and salt

¼ to ½ tsp cayenne pepper

1 large potato

¼ cup uncooked long-grain rice

2 small leeks

2 thin carrots, or 10 baby carrots

2 small peppers, preferably 1 red and 1 yellow

½ lb (250 g) firm-fleshed fish, such as grouper or sea bass

½ lb (250 g) medium-size shrimp, fresh or frozen

1 lb (500 g) mussels

½ lb (250 g) small scallops (optional)

½ cup coarsely chopped fresh basil or coriander

1. Heat 1 tablespoon of oil in a large saucepan set over low heat. Add garlic and sauté, stirring often, for 5 minutes. Add another tablespoon of oil. When oil is hot, sprinkle it with flour, then stir constantly for 2 minutes.

HONEY-GINGER GLAZED SALMON FOR TWO

Pour 1 cup orange juice into a frying pan. Stir in 2 teaspoons honey and 2 teaspoons grated fresh ginger or ½ teaspoon ground ginger. Bring to a boil. Add 2 salmon steaks, at least 1 inch thick. Cover and reduce heat so juice barely simmers. Cook 10 minutes, turning salmon halfway through cooking. Remove to a dinner plate. Boil sauce, uncovered, until reduced by half. Pour over salmon. *Serves 2.*

PER SERVING

Calories: 185

Protein: 16 g

Fat: 6 g

Carbohydrate: 17 g

Fiber: 2 g

Excellent source: Vitamin A, Vitamin C

Good source: Iron

2. Increase heat to medium. Gradually whisk in can of condensed chicken broth and 1 can of water or 2½ cups of chicken bouillon. Add clam juice and seasonings. Let mixture simmer, uncovered and whisking often, while preparing vegetables.

3. Peel potato only if the skin is thick. Cut into ⅓-inch cubes. Stir potato into simmering broth. Stir in rice. Cover and continue cooking. Slice off and discard about half of the dark green from the top of the leeks, tough outer leaves and root ends. Slice leeks in half lengthwise and spread outer leaves under cold running water to remove grit or sand. Slice leeks about ⅓ inch thick. Stir leeks into simmering broth. Thinly slice carrots and add to broth.

4. Cover and cook over medium-low heat until potatoes are almost tender, about 15 minutes. Stir often. Meanwhile, seed peppers and cut them into cubes. Slice fish into bite-size pieces. If shrimp are frozen, run cold water over them until all ice crystals are melted. Remove any shells but leave tails on. Scrub mussels under cold water and remove any beards.

5. When potatoes are almost tender, turn heat to high. Add peppers, fish and mussels, stirring until mixed. Cover and cook for 4 minutes. Stir in shrimp and scallops. Cover and continue cooking until mussels open and shrimp are bright pink, about 3 to 4 more minutes. Discard any mussels that haven't opened. Remove from the heat. Stir in the basil or coriander. Serve in large shallow soup bowls with warm garlic bread on the side. For a more substantial entrée, place a little cooked rice in the bottom of soup dishes and spoon gumbo over top.

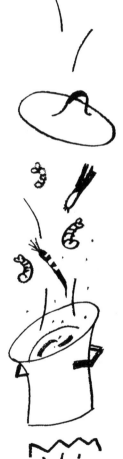

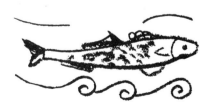

Roast Turkey à Deux

If you'd like to enjoy the company of someone special on a holiday weekend rather than spend your time cooking turkey for 20, here's our tantalizing recipe for fine dining à deux that will leave you lots of time for snuggling by the fire. And, as with all good turkey dinners, there'll be leftovers! This elegant dinner takes only 20 minutes to prepare. Just add a green vegetable, a good chilled chardonnay and cranberry sorbet or pumpkin ice cream for dessert.

PREPARATION TIME: 20 MINUTES
ROASTING TIME: 1 HOUR AND 30 MINUTES / MAKES: 2 SERVINGS

2½-lb (1.25-kg) bone-in turkey breast
1 cup apple juice
1 tsp dried rosemary
½ tsp dried leaf thyme
½ tsp poultry seasoning
¼ tsp salt
2 large baking potatoes, such as Yukon Gold, or small sweet potatoes
1 tbsp olive oil or melted butter

1. Preheat oven to 375°F (190°C). Remove skin from turkey only if you wish. Place turkey breast in a shallow glass baking dish just large enough to hold it. Pour apple juice over top, then sprinkle breast with seasonings. Tightly cover the pan with a piece of foil. Roast in center of oven for 1 hour.

2. As soon as turkey has been placed in oven, slice potatoes into wedges, about 1 inch wide. Put in a bowl and drizzle with oil. Toss until coated. Sprinkle with poultry seasoning and salt, tossing potatoes as you sprinkle on seasonings so they are evenly coated. Spread them out on a baking sheet. After turkey has been roasting 30 minutes, place baking sheet on bottom rack of oven and turn every 15 minutes until golden, about 1 hour for regular potatoes or 45 minutes for sweet potatoes.

MANDARIN CHRISTMAS SALSA
Finely chop 1 mandarin orange or tangerine and stir into ½ cup salsa along with ¼ cup finely chopped green pepper. Serve as a dip for large shrimp or nacho chips. *Makes ¾ cup.*

PER SERVING
WITHOUT SKIN

Calories: 407

Protein: 38 g

Fat: 8 g

Carbohydrate: 44 g

Fiber: 4 g

Excellent source: Vitamin C, Iron

3. After turkey has been roasting 1 hour, remove foil. Continue roasting, basting often, until turkey is golden, about 30 minutes more. Then, let it sit at room temperature, loosely covered with foil, for at least 10 minutes before slicing. Pour pan juices into a gravy boat to pour over slices. When you have sliced off the turkey you would like for dinner, immediately refrigerate the remainder. It will keep well refrigerated for at least 2 days, or can be frozen, then quickly defrosted in the microwave.

Rosé Pork Roast with Fall Vegetables

Anita Draycott, a superb editor and hostess, entertained us in her large comfortable kitchen with this outstanding roast. Rosé wine lends its delicate fruity taste to this one-dish oven dinner, complete with potatoes, squash and roasted apples. Serve the same rosé wine, well chilled, with dinner.

PREPARATION TIME: 20 MINUTES / BAKING TIME: 1½ HOURS

MAKES: 6 TO 8 SERVINGS

2- to 2½-lb (1- to 1.25-kg) center-cut pork loin roast
1 tsp each of dried rosemary, leaf thyme and oregano
1 tbsp olive oil
½ tsp each of salt and freshly ground black pepper
½ cup water
1 small squash, about 1 lb (500 g)
2 onions
4 large white potatoes or 2 large sweet potatoes
1 cup semi-dry rosé wine
4 crisp apples

HOLIDAY CRANBERRY CHÈVRE SPREAD

Whirl ¼ cup fresh or frozen cranberries and 1 tablespoon milk or orange juice in food processor until berries are coarsely chopped. Add a 5-oz (140-g) package creamy chèvre and process just until mixture is combined. Taste and add a generous pinch of sugar, if needed. Stir in ¼ cup finely chopped fresh coriander or parsley. Serve as a dip for zucchini spears, red pepper strips, snow peas, slices of pear and apple, or spread over thin slices of baguette. *Makes 1 cup.*

PER SERVING

Calories: 357
Protein: 24 g
Fat: 12 g
Carbohydrate: 38 g
Fiber: 5 g
Good source: Vitamin C, Iron

1. Preheat oven to 400°F (200°C). Make many shallow slits over surface of pork loin, especially through fat layer. Lightly crush rosemary with fingers. Mix oil with herbs, salt and pepper. Spread mixture over sides and top of roast, pressing a little of mixture into slits. Place roast in a large broiling pan or large roasting pan at least 12 x 14 inches (30 x 35 cm). Pour water around roast. Cover loosely with a large piece of foil. Bake in center of oven for 30 minutes.

2. Meanwhile, cut unpeeled squash into quarters. Seed squash, then slice into 1½-inch sections. Cut onions into quarters through root end. Scrub white potatoes and cut into quarters or peel and cut sweet potatoes into quarters.

3. When roast has cooked for 30 minutes, remove foil and scatter vegetables around meat. Sprinkle a little salt, pepper and rosemary over vegetables. Pour ½ cup wine over meat. Reduce heat to 350°F (180°C). Roast, uncovered, for 30 minutes, basting after 15 minutes. Meanwhile, core unpeeled apples and cut them into quarters.

4. After meat and vegetables have cooked together for 30 minutes, scatter apples around pork. Pour remaining ½ cup wine over pork. If vegetables and apples are crowded in pan, remove some of the vegetables to another pan. Pour a little wine over them. Basting often, continue roasting until apples and vegetables are golden-tipped, about 30 more minutes.

5. Remove roast to a cutting board, loosely cover with foil and let sit for at least 5 minutes before carving. Meanwhile, remove vegetables from pan and cover them to keep them warm. Skim off and discard any fat from pan juices. Whisk pan juices to stir up any browned bits. Slice pork and serve with roasted vegetables and apples, and pan juices.

NEW-STYLE SWEET 'N' SOUR GREENS

Wash a large bunch of green or red-tinged Swiss chard or kale or collard greens. Trim stems and leave on if you like. Slice leaves crosswise into 3 or 4 wide strips. Lightly coat a wide deep frying pan with olive oil. Add the greens and sauté until tender, about 5 minutes. Then toss with 2 tablespoons each of balsamic vinegar and brown sugar. *Serves 3 to 4.*

More Vitality Vegetables

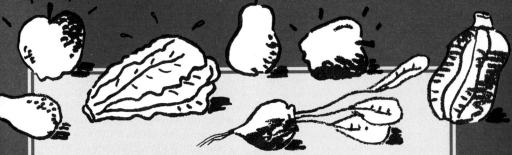

Asparagus in Garlic Vinaigrette with Chèvre

Great Garlicky Broccoli

Springtime Vegetable Roast

Glazed Turnip with Fresh Dill

New-Fashioned Brussels Sprouts

Sage 'n' Garlic Mashed Potatoes

Baked Vegetable Rustico

Vegetable Curry P.D.Q.

Roasted Vegetables

Curried Squash and Pepper Toss

Sensational Four Pepper Sauté

CAULIFLOWER WITH SPICED YOGURT

Trim 1 head of cauliflower and divide into large florets. Put in a large saucepan with 1 inch of hot water. Cover and boil gently over high heat until done as you like, about 5 minutes. Meanwhile, combine ½ cup plain yogurt or low-fat sour cream in a small saucepan with ½ teaspoon paprika and ½ teaspoon dried dillweed. Cook over low heat, stirring often, just until warm, about 2 minutes. Drain cauliflower and toss with sauce. *Serves 4.*

PER SERVING

Calories: 51

Protein: 2 g

Fat: 4 g

Carbohydrate: 4 g

Fiber: 1 g

Excellent source: Folic Acid

Asparagus in Garlic Vinaigrette with Chèvre

One shouldn't fool around a lot with asparagus. It's best simply steamed — but here's a delicious way to dress it up for company.

PREPARATION TIME: 5 MINUTES / MICROWAVING TIME: 4 MINUTES

MAKES: 4 SERVINGS

1 lb (500 g) asparagus, about 4 bunches
1 tbsp olive oil
2 tbsp red-wine vinegar or tarragon vinegar
1 crushed garlic clove
Generous pinches of dried leaf oregano and salt
Crumbled chèvre or feta cheese (optional)

1. Break tough ends off asparagus, usually about ½ inch, and discard them. Rinse spears under cold running water. On a pie plate, arrange spears with tips toward center and stems to outer edge, wagon-wheel style. Cover with waxed paper. Microwave on high until as tender as you like, about 4 to 6 minutes.

2. Meanwhile, whisk oil with vinegar, garlic, oregano and salt. Pour dressing over hot asparagus in pie plate. Turn spears until coated. Arrange them on a platter and sprinkle with cheese, if you like. Serve right away because the color of the asparagus may be dulled if it sits in the vinaigrette for more than an hour or two.

VEGETARIAN MAIN COURSES

Here's our line-up of vegetarian entrées.

Quesadillas with Ripe Mango, Chèvre and Coriander *(p. 12)*

Quick Curried Lentil and Carrot Soup (with vegetable broth) *(p. 36)*

Garden Veggie Lentil Salad *(p. 41)*

Healthy Greek Luncheon Salad *(p. 43)*

Shanghai Noodle Salad *(p. 69)*

Easy-Make, Easy-Eat Layered Pasta Bake *(p. 75)*

Mexican-Spiced Beans 'n' Rice *(p. 87)*

New-Style Easy Stuffed Peppers (see vegetarian variation) *(p. 89)*

Couscous with Stir-Fried Spring Vegetables *(p. 91)*

Vegetarian Mushroom and Red Pepper Cabbage Rolls *(p. 92)*

Lusty Vegetable Stew with Feta and Basil *(p. 94)*

Phyllo Vegetable Pie *(p. 104)*

Vegetable Curry P.D.Q. (with cashews) *(p. 120)*

Great Garlicky Broccoli

Bright green and slightly crunchy, this flavorful rendition of broccoli will give you one more easy way to serve this nutritional superstar! Broccoli, by the way, contains quite a bit of protein and this version is an excellent source of vitamin C and folic acid.

PREPARATION TIME: 10 MINUTES / COOKING TIME: 10 MINUTES

MAKES: 4 SERVINGS

1 large bunch broccoli
2 tsp olive oil
2 large crushed garlic cloves
¾ cup chicken broth or water
Pinches of salt and freshly ground black pepper
2 tbsp freshly grated Parmesan cheese

1. Cut broccoli florets from stalks, then separate them into bite-size pieces. Trim any tough outer portions from stalks, then slice into ½-inch rounds. Keep stalks and florets separate.

2. Heat oil, garlic, broth and seasonings in a large frying pan set over medium heat. When mixture is bubbling, add stalk pieces and cook, uncovered and stirring often, until about half of liquid has evaporated and stalks are almost tender, about 3 minutes. Toss in florets and increase heat to high. Stir-fry until florets are bright green and done as you like, about 4 to 5 more minutes. Sprinkle them with Parmesan and serve. Two tablespoons Parmesan is enough for flavor, but if you want to make this an entrée, top with additional cheese, or a dollop of light sour cream or yogurt.

BRAVO BROCCOLI

One cup of cooked broccoli supplies about a quarter of our daily requirement of vitamin A in the form of beta-carotene, more vitamin C than a glass of orange juice, 5 g of protein, as well as calcium, and folic acid — all for only 44 calories. It's great in a stir-fry, eaten raw in a salad, lightly blanched on a vegetable platter with a low-fat dip or simply steamed and seasoned with lemon, garlic, pepper and salt.

PER SERVING

Calories:	84
Protein:	7 g
Fat:	4 g
Carbohydrate:	8 g
Fiber:	3 g
Excellent source:	Vitamin C, Folic Acid
Good source:	Vitamin A

Springtime Vegetable Roast

This is a glorious-looking vegetable mélange to make for your first spring party or Easter weekend. The fresh basil gives it a wake-up taste. You can make it ahead of the party and serve hot, at room temperature or cold.

PREPARATION TIME: 15 MINUTES / ROASTING TIME: 20 MINUTES

MAKES: 6 ONE-CUP SERVINGS

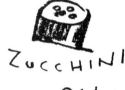

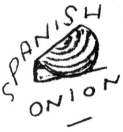

4 plum tomatoes
2 peppers, preferably red, yellow or orange
1 large sweet onion, such as Vidalia or Spanish
2 yellow summer squash
2 zucchini
8 tiny or 4 small new potatoes
2 tbsp olive oil
1 tbsp balsamic vinegar
3 crushed garlic cloves
½ tsp salt
¼ tsp freshly ground black pepper
¼ cup shredded fresh basil

1. Preheat oven to 425°F (220°C). Slice tomatoes in half. Holding each one over the sink, squeeze out all seeds and juice. Place them in a large mixing bowl, adding remaining vegetables as they are cut. Seed and cut peppers into long narrow triangles. Slice onion thickly and separate into rings. Slice squash and zucchini lengthwise into ½-inch-wide strips. Then cut them into bite-size pieces. Cut potatoes in half or quarters so they are no more than 1½ inches wide. Whisk oil with vinegar, garlic, salt and pepper. Drizzle over top of vegetables. Gently toss until vegetables are evenly coated.

PER SERVING

Calories: 162

Protein: 4 g

Fat: 5 g

Carbohydrate: 28 g

Fiber: 5 g

Excellent source: Vitamin C

Good source: Vitamin A, Folic Acid

2. Spread vegetables in a single layer on an ungreased baking sheet or roasting pan. Bake in center of oven, stirring twice, until vegetables are golden-tinged and just tender, about 20 minutes. Spoon into a heat-proof bowl. Sprinkle vegetables with basil, then gently toss. Serve warm or at room temperature. This is best on the day it's made but it's also good served the next day as a cold salad.

Glazed Turnip with Fresh Dill

Treat turnip to a mild sweet-and-sour glaze as a dress-up when presenting it with a golden roast turkey.

<u>PREPARATION TIME: 10 MINUTES / COOKING TIME: 15 MINUTES</u>
<u>MAKES: 4 SERVINGS</u>

1 medium-size turnip or large rutabaga
¼ tsp salt
2 tbsp granulated sugar
1 tbsp butter
1 tbsp white vinegar
2 tbsp chopped fresh dill, or ½ tsp dried dillweed
Pinches of salt and white pepper

1. Peel turnip, then cut it into bite-size strips, about 1½ inches x ½ inch. Cover turnip with boiling water in a saucepan. Add salt and 1 tablespoon sugar. Boil gently, partially covered, until just fork-tender, about 10 to 15 minutes. Drain it well but leave in saucepan.

2. Add butter. Sprinkle turnip with vinegar, remaining tablespoon of sugar, dill and generous pinches of salt and white pepper. Stir constantly over medium heat until turnip is lightly glazed, about 2 minutes. Serve right away or if making ahead, refrigerate. Cover when chilled and it will keep well for up to 1 day. Then, reheat in a saucepan over low heat or in the microwave.

FABULOUS FENNEL
Fennel root, with its white, bulbous bottom, may look like celery but actually tastes like licorice. Store fresh fennel, wrapped in plastic, in the refrigerator and use within 1 week. To serve, trim any brown parts from base. Cut coarse leaves from top or leave a few feathery fronds attached, if you like. Slice lengthwise into long strips for relish trays or crosswise into thin pieces for salads. Lightly steamed or sautéed until tender-crisp, fennel is also delightful as a hot vegetable. The seeds of mature plants are used to flavor sweet Italian sausage, tomato sauces and breads.

PER SERVING

Calories: 86	
Protein: 1 g	
Fat: 3 g	
Carbohydrate: 15 g	
Fiber: 2 g	
Good source: Vitamin C	

New-Fashioned Brussels Sprouts

Sautéed red onion gently tames assertive brussels sprouts and bacon adds a marvelous smoky taste. Prepare most of this appealing-looking dish ahead for a holiday dinner.

PREPARATION TIME: 10 MINUTES / COOKING TIME: 18 MINUTES
MAKES: 8 SERVINGS

1½ lbs (750 g) brussels sprouts, about 2 pints (1 L)
1 tbsp olive oil or butter, or 4 strips lean bacon
1 red onion, sliced into thin rings
1 tbsp freshly squeezed lemon juice
¼ tsp freshly ground black pepper
¼ tsp salt (optional)

1. Fill a large saucepan half full with hot water and bring it to a boil over high heat. Meanwhile, trim away tough stem ends from brussels sprouts and remove any discolored leaves. In stem end, cut an "X" about ¼ inch deep. This helps to speed up the cooking of the dense stem ends.

2. When water is boiling, add sprouts. Adjust heat so water continues to boil gently. Cook sprouts, uncovered, until almost tender, about 5 minutes. Then, drain them and rinse with cold water.

3. Heat oil in a large frying pan set over medium heat. Or, slice bacon into 1-inch pieces and sauté, stirring often, until some of the fat has collected in the pan, about 3 to 4 minutes. Add onion and cook, stirring often, until onion has softened, about 5 minutes. If using bacon, drain off most of the accumulated fat, leaving only about 1 tablespoon in pan with bacon pieces and onion.

4. Add drained sprouts, lemon juice and pepper. Continue cooking over medium heat, stirring often, until sprouts are hot, about 5 minutes. Taste and add salt, if you wish. Turn mixture into a heated serving dish.

MIGHTY SPROUTS

Brussels sprouts are one of the highest fiber vegetables. One-half cup cooked contains about 3.5 g, which makes a good dent in the 20 to 35 daily grams recommended. It also contains almost our daily supply of vitamin C as well as generous amounts of beta-carotene, vitamin B6, folic acid and smaller amounts of other nutrients — all for only about 30 calories. Cook in a small amount of boiling water until just tender. Overcooking reduces color and strengthens the flavor. To speed up cooking, cut a cross in the stem end.

PER SERVING

Calories: 65

Protein: 3 g

Fat: 2 g

Carbohydrate: 12 g

Fiber: 4 g

Excellent source: Vitamin C, Folic Acid

MAKE AHEAD: *Prepare recipe up to Step 4, but do not heat brussels sprouts with onion mixture. Simply turn onion mixture into a resealable bag. Place brussels sprouts in a separate bag. Refrigerate both for up to 1 day. Then, turn contents of both bags into a frying pan and cook according to Step 4 in recipe.*

Sage 'n' Garlic Mashed Potatoes

Give mashed potatoes a flavor boost with a touch of sweet garlic and sage. Then, beat them into creamy surrender with low-fat, high-flavor buttermilk instead of cream and butter. Perfect with any roast.

PREPARATION TIME: 20 MINUTES / COOKING TIME: 25 MINUTES

MAKES: 6 SERVINGS

2 lbs (1 kg) potatoes, about 6 medium potatoes
4 garlic cloves, peeled
1 tbsp butter or olive oil
1½ tsp finely chopped fresh sage, or ¼ tsp rubbed dried sage, crumbled
½ tsp salt
¼ tsp black or white pepper
½ cup buttermilk or light sour cream

1. Peel potatoes and cut them in half. Place them in a large saucepan along with whole garlic cloves. Cover potatoes with water. Place saucepan over medium-high heat and boil gently, partially covered, until potatoes are very tender, about 20 to 25 minutes. Drain well.

2. Mash garlic cloves with a fork. Then mash potatoes and garlic cloves together using a potato masher or by putting them through a food mill. Return potatoes to saucepan. Beat in remaining ingredients. If potatoes are not warm enough, cover saucepan and return to medium-low heat. Continue heating potatoes, stirring often, until they are as warm as you like. Taste and add more sage, if you wish.

INCREDIBLY CREAMY MASHED POTATOES

Slice 8 peeled potatoes in half and place in a large saucepan. Cover with water. Boil gently, partially covered, until very tender, about 20 to 30 minutes. Drain and mash. Beat in 2 tablespoons olive oil or butter, 1 cup light sour cream, 1 teaspoon salt and a pinch of pepper. Pile into heated serving dish. Can be kept warm in a 250°F (130°C) oven. *Serves 8.*

PER SERVING

Calories: 141	
Protein: 3 g	
Fat: 2 g	
Carbohydrate: 28 g	
Fiber: 2 g	

Baked Vegetable Rustico

This is a great party dish, partly because you simply chop all the vegetables, stir together and bake — no sautéing needed — and partly because it's an all-you-need side dish containing lots of veggies and potatoes. It's great hot, at room temperature or cold — so you can make it ahead for a party — and it also freezes well.

PREPARATION TIME: 15 MINUTES / BAKING TIME: 1½ HOURS
MAKES: 4 TO 6 SERVINGS

1 medium-size eggplant

2 large potatoes

2 large green peppers

1 large Spanish or red onion

2 medium-size zucchini

3 large tomatoes, or a 28-oz (796-mL) can plum tomatoes, well drained

8 garlic cloves, crushed, or 2 tbsp minced garlic

2 tbsp olive oil

2 tsp dried basil

1 tsp each of dried leaf oregano and salt

½ tsp each of ground black pepper and cayenne

1 tbsp sugar

2 tbsp balsamic vinegar

1. Peel eggplant and cut into 1-inch cubes. Put cubes in a large deep saucepan or casserole that will hold at least 16 cups (4 L). Cut unpeeled potatoes into ½-inch cubes, slice peppers into 1-inch pieces and finely chop onion. Add them to casserole. Slice zucchini lengthwise into quarters, then slice it into ½-inch pieces and add to other vegetables. Coarsely chop unpeeled tomatoes and add them along with any juices, or cut drained canned tomatoes into bite-size pieces and add.

SASSY SAUTÉED TOMATOES

Thickly slice 2 ripe tomatoes. Heat 2 teaspoons olive oil in a frying pan set over medium-high heat. Add tomatoes. Sprinkle with generous pinches of dried basil or chopped fresh basil, cayenne pepper, salt, freshly ground black pepper and granulated sugar. Sauté for about 2 minutes per side. Serve hot. Great with pita for sopping up the juices. *Serves 4.*

PER SERVING

Calories:	198
Protein:	5 g
Fat:	5 g
Carbohydrate:	37 g
Fiber:	7 g

Excellent source: Vitamin C

Good source: Vitamin A, Folic Acid, Iron

2. Preheat oven to 375°F (190°C). In a small bowl, stir garlic with oil and all seasonings. Add mixture to casserole and stir vigorously until vegetables are evenly coated.

3. Place casserole in oven and bake, uncovered, for 1½ hours. Stir at least every half hour. Vegetables at the top will appear to dry out but will actually take on a little roasted taste. Baking uncovered also allows some vegetable juices to evaporate, and concentrated vegetable juices will be soaked up by eggplant and zucchini.

4. Remove hot casserole from oven. Sprinkle mixture with sugar. Drizzle in vinegar and stir until well mixed. Taste. You may want to add more salt, sugar or vinegar. It's wonderful sprinkled with lots of chopped fresh basil, coriander or parsley.

GREAT ADDITION: *Stir together ½ cup chopped parsley, 3 cloves minced fresh garlic and the finely grated peel of 1 lemon, then sprinkle over top of hot casserole just before serving.*

MAKE AHEAD: *Bake casserole completely. Remove from oven, cover and let sit until it reaches room temperature, then refrigerate or freeze. Refrigerated, it will keep well for 3 to 4 days. Taste before serving. You may need to stir in a little minced fresh garlic, chopped fresh or dried basil or a drizzle of balsamic vinegar to freshen up flavor before serving. If you want to reheat, small amounts reheat beautifully in the microwave on medium power. Or reheat in a 350°F (180°C) oven in a covered dish. Freeze in resealable plastic bags in serving-size amounts; you can quickly defrost in the microwave.*

DILLED ORANGE CARROTS

Peel 4 large carrots and slice into julienne strips. Put in a microwave-safe dish. Toss with 2 tablespoons orange juice and ½ teaspoon dried dillweed. Cover and microwave on high until carrots are tender, about 6 minutes. Add salt and pepper to taste. If you have fresh dill, omit the dried dillweed and stir about 2 tablespoons of chopped fresh dill into the cooked carrots. *Serves 2.*

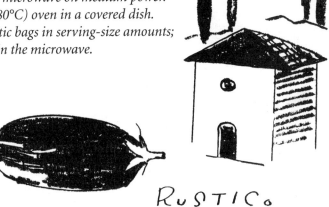

RuSTICo

Vegetable Curry P.D.Q.

A robust vegetable curry can be quick and easy. Makes a terrific side dish for chicken or veggie burgers, or add cashews and it's a complete main course.

PREPARATION TIME: 10 MINUTES / COOKING TIME: 15 MINUTES
MAKES: 4 SERVINGS

GREENS AND SHALLOTS

Rinse 1 large bunch Swiss chard or 2 bunches of spinach with cold water to remove all grit. Slice chard into 2-inch wide pieces. Remove tough stems from spinach. Heat 1 tablespoon olive oil in a large wide saucepan. Add 2 tablespoons finely chopped shallots or 2 teaspoons minced garlic. Stir over medium-low heat for 5 minutes. Add enough greens to about half fill the pan. Turn heat to medium-high. Stir almost constantly. Add remaining greens as soon as there is room in the pan. Stir until chard is tender or spinach is hot. Season with salt and pepper to taste. *Serves 4.*

1 large onion
2 jalapeño peppers, seeded, or ½ tsp crushed hot chilies
2 tsp olive oil or butter
2 crushed cloves garlic, or 1 tbsp bottled minced garlic
2 tsp curry powder
1 medium-size cauliflower
4 large ripe tomatoes
½ cup light sour cream
Toasted cashews or sesame seeds (optional)

1. Coarsely chop onion and finely chop jalapeño peppers. Heat oil in a wide frying pan. Add onion, garlic and hot peppers. Sprinkle mixture with curry powder. Sauté over low heat for 5 minutes, stirring often.

2. Meanwhile, break cauliflower into florets and slice the thick base. Quarter tomatoes, then slice wedges in half. Add cauliflower and tomatoes to sautéing onions. Turn heat to medium high and stir frequently until cauliflower is done as you like and a sauce has formed, about 10 to 15 minutes. Stir in sour cream and serve curry over rice. For a complete vegetarian entrée, sprinkle each serving with ¼ cup toasted cashews or 2 tablespoons sesame seeds.

PER SERVING

Calories: 143	
Protein: 7 g	
Fat: 5 g	
Carbohydrate: 22 g	
Fiber: 6 g	
Excellent source: Vitamin A, Vitamin C, Folic Acid	

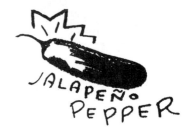
JALAPEÑO PEPPER

Roasted Vegetables

*Serve a big platter of sturdy root vegetables roasted to
a golden sweetness with any roasted dinner, from
roast beef to Sunday chicken.*

PREPARATION TIME: 20 MINUTES / ROASTING TIME: 30 MINUTES

MAKES: 6 SERVINGS

1 lb (500 g) potatoes, about 3 medium sweet or
  white potatoes

6 carrots

6 parsnips, or 1 large turnip

1 butternut or pepper squash

1 large red or Spanish onion

2 to 3 tbsp balsamic vinegar

2 tbsp olive oil

1 tsp dried rosemary, crumbled

½ tsp each of sugar and salt

¼ tsp freshly ground black pepper

1. Preheat oven to 450°F (230°C). Peel sweet potatoes. Peel white potatoes if you wish. Cut sweet or white
potatoes into wedges. Peel carrots, parsnips, squash and
onion. Seed squash and cut vegetables into 1½-inch
chunks. In a large bowl, stir vinegar with remaining
ingredients. (If you love balsamic vinegar, use 3 tablespoons.) Add vegetables and toss until they are coated.

2. Spread vegetables out, in a single layer, in a large
roasting pan or on 2 large baking sheets. Bake in center
of oven, stirring often, until potatoes are golden and
tender, about 30 to 45 minutes.

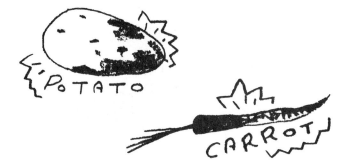

FREEZING VEGGIES

Vegetables that are usually
eaten raw do not freeze
well because they can
become mushy or limp on
thawing. Tomatoes and
celery, however, can be
frozen for use in soups
and stews. Eggplant
becomes watery and
darkens in color. Corn
on the cob has a greater
tendency than other
vegetables to develop
off-flavors during frozen
storage but this problem
can be avoided by
blanching for the
recommended times.
Asparagus, green and
wax beans, peas, spinach,
whole kernel corn and
mashed cooked squash
are good candidates for
freezing.

PER SERVING

Calories: 336

Protein: 6 g

Fat: 5 g

Carbohydrate: 72 g

Fiber: 13 g

Excellent source: Vitamin A,
Vitamin C, Folic Acid

Good source: Calcium, Iron

SQUASH ALMIGHTY

HUBBARD

Rounded with a tapered end, hubbards can grow to watermelon size. Their wrinkled hard skin can be dark-green, blue-gray or orange-colored. Generally dry, the pale yellowish-orange flesh tastes fairly sweet. Choose medium-size hubbards for the best taste.

• Bake unpeeled halves, cut-side down, with a little water in a 375°F (190°C) oven until tender, at least 45 minutes. Or, boil or steam peeled cubes for about 30 minutes.

• Mash squash and jazz it up with butter, maple syrup or brown sugar. Cube squash and toss with sliced green onions, grated orange peel, ground cinnamon, ginger or poultry seasoning. Moisten with orange juice or sesame oil.

TURBAN

Easy to identify, this squash's flattened round base topped with three knobs resembles a colorful orange turban and makes a great table decoration. Its yellow to orange-colored flesh has a rich full taste.

• Pierce squash and cook whole in microwave on high for 8 to 12 minutes. Discard seeds and scoop out flesh. Mash squash and stir with green onions or cube squash and spice with curry or mix with wild rice and nuts for a pilaf, then serve in hollowed-out shell.

BUTTERNUT

Pear-shaped with a bulbous end, butternut squash has a smooth dull-beige skin. Its bright orange flesh has an equally rich sweet taste.

• To make the hard shell easier to cut, microwave squash on high for 2 minutes, then slice in half or rings for baking. Peel baked squash and glaze as you would sweet potatoes. Or, add raw cubes to stewed tomato mixture, soups and stews. Very good in black bean or lentil soups.

SPAGHETTI SQUASH

Resembling a small yellow football, the spaghetti squash shell is not hard. When cooked, the stringy-yellow interior separates into long "spaghetti-like" strands. Very mild and slightly sweet-tasting, it makes a great "low-cal" stand-in for pasta and it's a good source of vitamin A and potassium.

• Bake at 375°F (190°C) for 50 to 60 minutes. Or, pierce and microwave on high for 12 to 15 minutes. Let stand 5 minutes. Slice in half. Scoop out seeds. Use a fork to scrape strands from shell. If all the strands won't come away from shell, return to microwave. Toss with tomato sauce, olive oil and herbs or Parmesan and green onions.

GOLDEN NUGGET

This squash looks like a tiny, bright-orange pumpkin with stand-out ridges instead of grooves. Although mainly used as a decoration, its intense orange flesh has a slightly sweet squash taste.

• These small squash bake quickly in the oven or microwave. Or, steam halves or quarters for about 20 minutes. Enjoy with butter and brown sugar, maple syrup or honey. Good filled with poultry stuffing.

ACORN OR PEPPER

Acorn-shaped with deeply ribbed smooth shell, this squash now comes in dark green, bright yellow or white. The flesh is mild, fairly sweet and pale yellow to orange in color.

• Slice in half and bake at 375°F (190°C) up to 45 minutes or microwave on high 8 to 12 minutes. Perfect for glazing or stuffing with meat or rice fillings.

Curried Squash and Pepper Toss

A pretty and unusual combo that's highly flavored. Perfect as a veggie entrée sprinkled liberally with good-quality Parmesan or as a harvest partner for pork chops or roast chicken.

PREPARATION TIME: 15 MINUTES / COOKING TIME: 25 MINUTES

MAKES: 4 SERVINGS

1 tbsp olive oil or butter
¼ cup water
1 large onion, thinly sliced
2 crushed garlic cloves
1 tbsp curry powder
2 large ripe tomatoes
4 cups bite-size pieces of squash, such as butternut or acorn
¼ tsp salt
1 large green pepper

1. Heat oil and water in a wide saucepan set over medium heat. Separate onion into rings and add them to pan along with garlic. Sprinkle mixture with curry powder and cook, stirring often, until water has evaporated, about 2 minutes.

2. Coarsely chop tomatoes. Do not seed them. When onion is fairly soft, stir in squash and tomatoes, along with any tomato juice and seeds. Stir in salt.

3. Cover, reduce heat to low and cook for 15 minutes, stirring often. Seed pepper, cut into bite-size pieces and stir into mixture. Continue cooking until done as you like, about 5 more minutes.

PEPPER TOSS

KOHLRABI: THREE TASTES IN ONE

Kohlrabi has a rather unique appearance and can liven up any meal. Although it belongs to the cabbage family, it has a bulbous stem with leaves that resemble those of a turnip. It has a crisp texture with a mild flavor. When served raw, it tastes like a radish. Steamed, boiled or microwaved, it has a delicate taste that's a cross between a cabbage and a turnip.

PER SERVING

Calories:	142
Protein:	3 g
Fat:	4 g
Carbohydrate:	28 g
Fiber:	5 g
Excellent source:	Vitamin A, Vitamin C
Good source:	Folic Acid, Iron

Sensational Four Pepper Sauté

A smart idea inspired by Lorraine Greey. We guarantee this will be the most colorful vegetable sauté you've ever done.

PREPARATION TIME: 20 MINUTES / COOKING TIME: 25 MINUTES
MAKES: 6 TO 8 SERVINGS

1 large onion, peeled
1 tbsp olive or vegetable oil
6 crushed garlic cloves
4 to 6 sweet green peppers
2 sweet yellow or orange peppers
2 banana peppers
2 jalapeño peppers, seeded and finely chopped, or 1 tsp hot red pepper flakes
¼ tsp salt
2 large ripe tomatoes

1. Slice onion in half. Place it cut-side down on cutting board and thinly slice. Heat oil in a large wide frying pan over medium heat. Add the onion and garlic. Sauté, stirring often, until soft, at least 10 minutes. Add a little water, up to ¼ cup, if necessary.

2. Meanwhile, seed sweet and banana peppers and slice into strips, about ⅓-inch thick. Finely chop jalapeño peppers. When onions are soft, add all the peppers and salt.

3. Sauté, stirring often, for 10 minutes. Coarsely chop tomatoes. Stir them in and continue sautéing for 2 to 3 more minutes, until they are hot. Turn into a pretty dish and serve hot, at room temperature or chilled.

PUMPKIN POWER

Cook small pumpkins in microwave. Or, place a 2-lb (1-kg) slice in a 400°F (200°C) oven for 5 minutes to soften. Remove skin and cut into cubes. Toss 2 cups of cubes with 2 tablespoons vegetable oil, a pinch of salt and pepper. Spread out in an oven dish and roast until tender, about 25 minutes. Serve with pork or chicken. Or bake pumpkin, then purée pulp and freeze or use right away to make pies, muffins, soups, etc.

PER SERVING

Calories: 60

Protein: 2 g

Fat: 2 g

Carbohydrate: 11 g

Fiber: 3 g

Excellent source: Vitamin C

Good source: Vitamin A

Fabulous Finales

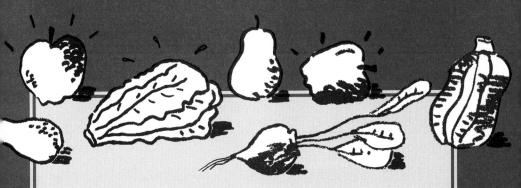

Tropical Fruit Flambé

Caramelized Maple Tofu with Fresh Berries

Tangy Lemon-Yogurt Cake

Fresh Mint, Mango and Berry Salad

Easy Chocolate-Banana Bread

Carrot Tropicale Cake

Smart Satisfying Brownies

Dream Cake

Fresh Strawberry Rhubarb Sauce

Sedated Strawberries

Ultimate Summer Fruit Salad

Tropical Fruit Flambé

Mangoes, rum and island heat add up to a sophisticated finale for any meal.

PREPARATION TIME: 10 MINUTES / COOKING TIME: 6 MINUTES
MAKES: 4 SERVINGS

FRESH BERRY AND ORANGE SALSA

Hull and slice 1 pint (500 mL) strawberries into quarters. Mix with 1 coarsely chopped orange and 1 green-skinned apple. Toss with 1 to 2 tablespoons granulated sugar, 1 to 2 teaspoons lemon juice and 1 teaspoon grated fresh ginger. Serve with frozen yogurt, ice cream or at brunch on its own. Salsa is best served the same day it is made. *Makes 3 cups.*

1 ripe mango
2 ripe but firm bananas
2 cups strawberries (optional)
1 to 2 tbsp butter
½ cup brown sugar
Pinches each of cinnamon and salt
3 tbsp rum, preferably dark

1. Peel and cut mango into bite-size pieces. Peel and diagonally slice bananas into ½-inch pieces. Stem berries. Slice them in half. Measure out all remaining ingredients and place close to cooking area before starting.

2. Just before serving, melt butter in a large non-stick frying pan set over medium heat. Stir in brown sugar, cinnamon and salt. Cook, without stirring, until entire mixture is bubbling, about 2 minutes. Stir in mango.

3. Cook, stirring often, until juices from mango form a sauce, then stir in bananas and berries. Immediately warm rum on high in the microwave for 30 seconds or heat in a very small saucepan set over medium heat just until it feels warm to the touch. Do not let it bubble. Immediately pour rum over hot fruit and set it alight with a match. Serve immediately over frozen yogurt or ice cream or use as a filling for crêpes.

PER SERVING

Calories:	232
Protein:	1 g
Fat:	3 g
Carbohydrate:	49 g
Fiber:	2 g
Good source:	Vitamin A

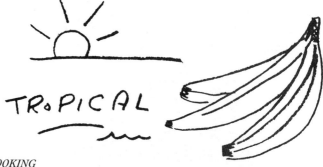

TROPICAL

Caramelized Maple Tofu with Fresh Berries

Chef James Saunders from Muskoka's Sherwood Inn nabbed first place in the annual Ducane Barbecue Contest with this innovative grilled dessert. Tofu rarely appeals to us but this version tastes like crème caramel — yet it's made with only healthy tofu soaked in maple syrup, grilled until warm, surrounded with berries, then moistened with fresh orange and lemon juices.

PREPARATION TIME: 20 MINUTES / REFRIGERATION TIME: OVERNIGHT
GRILLING TIME: 6 MINUTES / MAKES: 4 TO 8 SERVINGS

1 lb (500 g) piece of extra-firm tofu
½ cup maple syrup
1 pint fresh strawberries, about 2 cups, hulled
   and sliced
Balsamic vinegar (optional)
1 orange
1 lime

1. Cut block of tofu horizontally into 2 or 3 large slices, about ½ inch thick. Put them in a container that is not much larger than the tofu. Pour maple syrup over top. Refrigerate, preferably overnight, to give tofu a chance to soak up the maple syrup. If tofu is not covered by maple syrup, turn slices halfway through the marinating time.

2. When you're ready to grill, place tofu on an oiled grill and barbecue just until warm, about 3 to 4 minutes per side. Gently turn slices with a wide spatula. Place them on a dessert plate. Toss berries with a spritz of balsamic vinegar. Arrange them around warm tofu. Squeeze a little orange juice and lime juice over tofu and serve.

MAPLE RHUBARB SAUCE

Put 4 cups of fresh or frozen rhubarb, cut into 1-inch pieces, in a saucepan with 2 tablespoons water and ½ teaspoon ground cinnamon. Cover and cook over medium-low heat, stirring often, until fruit is soft, about 7 minutes. Stir in 2 tablespoons each of maple syrup and brown sugar. Serve warm in dessert dishes or spoon around ice cream or frozen yogurt. *Serves 4.*

PER SERVING

Calories: 117

Protein: 9 g

Fat: 1 g

Carbohydrate: 19 g

Fiber: 3 g

Good source: Vitamin C

Tangy Lemon-Yogurt Cake

Yogurt and fresh lemon juice give this cake a refreshing natural lemon flavor, and the yogurt gives low-fat richness and a hit of calcium.

PREPARATION TIME: 20 MINUTES / BAKING TIME: 35 MINUTES

MAKES: 10 TO 12 WEDGES

1 large lemon

1 cup plain 2% yogurt

2½ cups cake-and-pastry flour

2 tsp baking powder

½ tsp baking soda

½ tsp salt

½ cup butter, at room temperature

1 cup granulated sugar

1 egg, beaten

2 tsp vanilla

Icing sugar

6 cups mixed berries, such as sliced strawberries, raspberries and blueberries

1. Preheat oven to 350°F (180°C). Grease a 9½-inch (24-cm) springform pan or coat it with nonstick cooking spray, then lightly flour. Finely grate peel from lemon and squeeze out juice. You should have ⅓ cup lemon juice. Stir lemon peel and juice into yogurt. Measure flour, baking powder, baking soda and salt into a mixing bowl. Stir with a fork until evenly combined.

2. In a large mixing bowl, using an electric mixer, beat butter on medium-high speed until creamy, about 3 minutes. While beating, gradually add sugar, then egg and vanilla until well blended.

3. Using a spatula, stir half of flour mixture into butter mixture just until combined. Then, stir in half of yogurt mixture, stirring just until combined. Repeat with remaining flour and yogurt, stirring just until combined. Batter will be thick.

YOGURT — KEEP IT PLAIN

Plain yogurt has twice as much calcium as cottage cheese — about 380 mg per cup compared to 150 mg in a cup of cottage cheese. Fruit-bottomed yogurts, however, are less nutritious than plain since the fruit takes up space in the cup, giving you less yogurt, calcium and other important nutrients.

PER WEDGE

Calories: 269

Protein: 4 g

Fat: 9 g

Carbohydrate: 44 g

Fiber: 3 g

Good source: Vitamin C

4. Pour into prepared springform pan and smooth top. Bake in center of oven until a cake tester inserted into center comes out clean, about 35 to 40 minutes. Let cake cool on a rack for 5 minutes before removing springform sides. This cake is best served the same day it is made. However, covered and refrigerated, it will keep well for several days or in the freezer for several months. Defrost cake completely before unwrapping. Serve wedges sprinkled with icing sugar and topped with mixed berries. It's also good as a snacking cake.

Fresh Mint, Mango and Berry Salad

While there may be health in every bite, it's the refreshing alliance and gorgeous look that makes this a three-star winner.

PREPARATION TIME: 15 MINUTES / MAKES: 7 SERVINGS

½ ripe honeydew melon, peeled

1 ripe mango

1 pint strawberries, about 2 cups

2 tbsp freshly squeezed lemon juice

¼ cup coarsely chopped fresh mint, or
   ½ tsp dried mint

Pinch of salt

2 tbsp granulated sugar (optional)

Cottage cheese or crumbled chèvre, feta or
   blue cheese (optional)

1. Remove seeds from melon. Cut melon into bite-size cubes and place them in a large bowl. Slice peel from mango. Cut pulp away from stone and cube pulp. Add to melon cubes. Depending on their size, halve or quarter berries. Add to fruit mixture and gently toss.

2. Stir in lemon juice, mint and salt. Taste and add sugar, if needed. If serving as a main course or appetizer, however, skip sugar and serve over cottage cheese or on a bed of greens with a little chèvre crumbled over top.

BEAUTIFUL BERRIES
A cup of most berries contains about as much fiber as two slices of whole wheat bread and less than 100 calories. Avoid buying moldy or crushed berries. Pick through the berries and discard any soft ones before refrigerating. It's best to wash and sort berries just before serving as washing them before refrigerating speeds up spoilage.

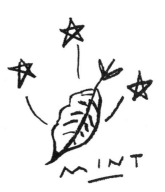

PER SERVING

Calories: 68	
Protein: 1 g	
Fat: Trace	
Carbohydrate: 18 g	
Fiber: 2 g	
Excellent source: Vitamin C	
Good source: Folic Acid	

BETH'S BANANA CREAM

Beth Currie, a superb Toronto hostess and cook, gave us the idea of topping a refreshing party fruit salad with healthy banana cream instead of rich whipping cream. Beth purées 2 ripe bananas with 2 tablespoons honey, then drizzles purée over a salad of strawberries, sliced kiwis, pears and red and green seedless grapes.

MELON AND BLUEBERRY COMPOTE

Peel and seed a cantaloupe and a honeydew melon. Cut pulp into bite-size pieces and put in a bowl. Stir in 2 cups blueberries, the finely grated peel of 1 orange, ½ cup orange juice, 2 tablespoons rum and 1 teaspoon sugar. Refrigerate until cold. *Serves 6 to 8.*

PER WEDGE

Calories: 172

Protein: 3 g

Fat: 5 g

Carbohydrate: 31 g

Fiber: 2 g

Easy Chocolate-Banana Cake

What could possibly be better than banana bread? Lavell Baldock gave us the answer with this incredibly easy chocolate version we discovered in her husband Frank Baldock's Wine Express Newsletter. *She serves it on a sauce of puréed mango, topped with yogurt. Remember this cake is not only low-fat, but bursting with potassium-rich bananas.*

PREPARATION TIME: 15 MINUTES / BAKING TIME: 45 MINUTES
MAKES: 12 WEDGES

1½ cups all-purpose flour

½ cup granulated sugar

2 tbsp unsweetened cocoa

½ tsp each of baking powder and baking soda

¾ tsp salt

¼ tsp freshly grated or ground nutmeg

2 squares (2 oz/56 g) bittersweet baking chocolate, or 1 square each of semi-sweet and unsweetened chocolate

3 tbsp olive or vegetable oil

3 large bananas

¼ cup milk

1 egg, beaten

1½ tsp vanilla

1. Preheat oven to 350°F (180°C). Coat a 9-inch (23-cm) round or 8-inch (20-cm) square cake pan with cooking spray. In a large bowl using a fork, stir flour with sugar, cocoa, baking powder, baking soda, salt and nutmeg until blended. Break chocolate into chunks and place in a glass measuring cup with oil. Microwave on high for 1 minute. Stir until smooth.

2. Using a fork, mash bananas. Measure out 1½ cups and place in a medium-size bowl. Stir in milk, egg and vanilla until smooth. Then stir in oil-chocolate mixture.

3. Make a well in the center of dry ingredients. Pour banana-chocolate mixture into well. Stir just until evenly mixed. Immediately pour batter into prepared pan.

4. Bake in center of oven until a cake tester inserted in center right to the bottom comes out clean, about 45 minutes. Set pan on a rack and cool for 5 minutes. Turn out and serve warm, surrounded by a purée of mangoes or canned peaches, or topped with a dollop of yogurt and a sprinkling of fresh berries. Store, covered, at room temperature for 1 day, in refrigerator up to 4 days, or freeze.

Carrot Tropicale Cake

This healthy take on carrot cake came to us many years ago from Roz Abrams, a Montreal baker. We've used it over the years and even managed to reduce the fat and use healthy olive oil. The natural bran adds lots of fiber and texture, making it a perfect snack or breakfast cake. You don't even need an electric mixer — a fork works well.

PREPARATION TIME: 10 MINUTES / BAKING TIME: 40 MINUTES
MAKES: 16 SLICES

3 cups whole wheat or all-purpose flour
2 cups natural wheat bran
1 cup light brown sugar
2 tbsp baking powder
½ tsp baking soda
½ tsp salt
1½ tsp cinnamon
¼ tsp allspice
Pinch of ground cloves
1 cup golden raisins (optional)
14-oz (398-mL) can pineapple dessert tidbits
3 cups grated carrots
3 eggs
⅓ cup olive oil
1 cup buttermilk

CREAM CHEESE AND HONEY ICING

This is a light icing from cookbook author Nettie Cronish. Put 6 oz cream cheese (at room temperature), 2 tablespoons honey, 2 tablespoons orange juice and ¾ teaspoon vanilla in a bowl. Beat with an electric mixer or wooden spoon until creamy. Spread over cake. *Makes enough for a 9x13-inch (3.5-L) cake.*

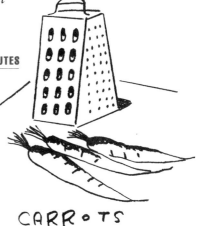

CARROTS

PER SLICE

Calories: 229	
Protein: 6 g	
Fat: 6 g	
Carbohydrate: 42 g	
Fiber: 7 g	
Excellent source: Vitamin A	
Good source: Iron	

1. Preheat oven to 350°F (180°C). Grease and flour a 10-inch (25-cm) tube or Bundt pan or a 9 x 13-inch (3-L) pan. Set aside. Measure flour, bran, brown sugar, baking powder, baking soda, salt and spices into a large bowl. Stir with a fork until blended. Stir in raisins. Set aside. Prepare pineapple by draining juice and saving it. Chop pineapple. Grate 3 cups carrots and set aside.

2. Measure eggs, oil and buttermilk into a large mixing bowl. Beat together until blended. Beat in ½ cup pineapple juice. Stir in dry ingredients. Finally, stir in pineapple and carrots just until mixed.

3. Turn into prepared pan and smooth the top. Bake in center of the oven for 40 to 45 minutes for a rectangular pan or 55 to 60 minutes for the Bundt pan. Cool on a rack for 10 minutes. Then turn out, if you wish, and cool completely. When cake is cool, dust the top with icing sugar or spread with Cream Cheese and Honey Icing. Covered and refrigerated, it will keep well for 4 or 5 days and freezes well.

FIBER-RICH

If you want to increase your fiber intake, check out the following fiber-rich recipes.

Smart Satisfying Brownies

The smart thing about these amazingly rich, decadent-tasting brownies is they need only a little olive oil — nutrient-rich applesauce adds moistness.

PREPARATION TIME: 15 MINUTES / BAKING TIME: 35 MINUTES

MAKES: 16 SQUARES

1½ cups all-purpose flour

¾ cup unsweetened cocoa

1½ cups granulated sugar

1 tsp baking powder

2 eggs

1 cup unsweetened store-bought applesauce

3 tbsp olive oil

1 tsp vanilla

1. Preheat oven to 350°F (180°C). Grease or coat with cooking spray an 8-inch (2-L) square baking dish. In a medium-size bowl, stir flour with cocoa, sugar and baking powder. In a large mixing bowl, beat eggs until blended. Stir in applesauce, oil and vanilla. When mixture is smooth, stir in flour mixture.

2. Turn into greased pan and smooth top. Bake in center of oven until edges begin to pull away from the sides and center seems firm when touched, about 35 minutes. Cool on a rack, then cut into squares. Brownies will keep well at room temperature for up to 1 day. For longer storage, cover tightly and freeze.

JUICE KNOW-HOW

Fruit "drinks", "sodas", "beverages", "punches", "blends", "sparklers", "ades" or "cocktails" may be mostly water, sugars and syrups. Look for 100% pure fruit juices for the maximum nutrition. Blends or drinks can be less than 50% pure fruit. Read the ingredients label and remember that items are listed in order of weight from heaviest to lightest. If juice is listed before water and/or corn syrup, you are probably getting a higher percentage of real fruit juice.

SPECIAL DRINKS

A scoop of frozen yogurt, glass of milk, banana and 6 to 8 strawberries whirled in the blender make a great after-school snack. A handful of blueberries turns it a horrible purple that most kids love!

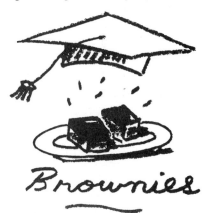

Brownies

PER SQUARE

Calories:	167
Protein:	3 g
Fat:	4 g
Carbohydrate:	31 g
Fiber:	2 g

Dream Cake

We've decided to call this old-fashioned mile-high light angel food cake "a dream cake" because it's made entirely without added fat or liquid yet it's moist and satisfying. Add cocoa to the batter if you've been craving chocolate, or top cake with a strawberry rhubarb sauce, sliced fresh berries or sliced mangoes and blueberries moistened with lime juice.

PREPARATION TIME: 20 MINUTES / BAKING TIME: 40 MINUTES
MAKES: 16 SLICES

1 cup cake-and-pastry flour
½ cup granulated sugar
¼ cup cocoa (optional)
1½ cups egg whites, from about 10 large eggs
1½ tsp cream of tartar
½ tsp salt
1 tsp vanilla
½ cup granulated sugar
Sliced fresh strawberries, raspberries and blueberries, or Fresh Strawberry Rhubarb Sauce* (see opposite page)

1. Preheat oven to 350°F (180°C). Place flour in a bowl. Add ½ cup sugar and cocoa. Stir until blended.

2. Combine egg whites, cream of tartar, salt and vanilla in a large mixing bowl. Using an electric mixer, beat at high speed until mixture will form soft peaks when beaters are lifted, about 3 minutes. Continuing to beat at high speed, gradually sprinkle in ½ cup sugar.

3. Hold a small sieve over egg white batter. Put about a quarter of flour mixture in sieve. Sprinkle it over batter. Using a wide spatula, gently fold flour mixture into batter. Repeat with remaining flour mixture. Immediately turn batter into an ungreased 10-inch (25-cm) tube pan. Gently smooth top. Bake in center of oven for 40 to 45 minutes or until cake springs back when lightly touched. Invert cake and cool in pan.

SMART RASPBERRY STORAGE

Raspberries are very delicate. So to avoid crushing, spread them out in a shallow container or on a cookie sheet. Cover loosely and refrigerate, or place sheets in freezer. When they are firm, pack into resealable plastic bags. One cup contains only 60 calories and is an excellent source of vitamin C.

PER SLICE
WITH HALF CUP SAUCE

Calories: 204

Protein: 4 g

Fat: Trace

Carbohydrate: 48 g

Fiber: 3 g

Excellent source: Vitamin C

4. When cool, loosen edges and remove cake from pan. Serve wedges of cake with a scattering of berries or Fresh Strawberry Rhubarb Sauce. Cake is best served within a day or 2 but will keep well in the refrigerator for at least 4 or 5 days and freezes well.

You will need a triple batch of Fresh Strawberry Rhubarb Sauce if you plan to serve the entire cake at one time.

Fresh Strawberry Rhubarb Sauce

We've teamed rhubarb's fleshy stalks with sweet berries for a luscious high-taste, slightly tangy sauce — perfect for spooning over angel food cake, shortcakes or as a breakfast eye-opener with yogurt.

PREPARATION TIME: 10 MINUTES
MICROWAVING TIME: 11 MINUTES / MAKES: 2½ CUPS

2 cups fresh or frozen rhubarb pieces
½ cup granulated sugar
2 tbsp cornstarch
1 pint (500 mL) strawberries

1. Cut rhubarb into ½-inch pieces. There's no need to defrost frozen rhubarb. When rhubarb is cut, measure out 2 cups. Put it in a microwave-safe dish that will hold about 8 cups (2 L). In another dish, stir sugar and cornstarch together with a fork until evenly blended. Stir sugar mixture into rhubarb.

2. Cover dish with a lid or plastic wrap vented in one corner. Microwave on high for 6 minutes if using fresh rhubarb or 8 minutes if rhubarb is frozen. Meanwhile wash, dry and hull berries. Cut them in half or quarters if they are large. You should have 2 to 2½ cups.

3. After rhubarb has cooked 6 or 8 minutes, stir in berries. Continue microwaving, uncovered and stirring once, until bubbling and thickened, about 3 minutes. Serve warm or refrigerate and serve cold. Covered and refrigerated, sauce will keep well for 2 days.

STRAWBERRIES

One cup provides more vitamin C than other berries — 89 mg, more than 100% of your daily requirement. Take advantage of summer harvest bargains by freezing your own: spread berries on a baking sheet and freeze until firm, then transfer to plastic bags. Fresh or frozen strawberries make a delicious pancake topping if you put them in a saucepan with a small amount of sugar, mash slightly, add a small amount of water, if necessary, and heat just until the sugar dissolves in the juice.

PER HALF CUP

Calories: 119	
Protein: 1 g	
Fat: Trace	
Carbohydrate: 30 g	
Fiber: 2 g	
Excellent source: Vitamin C	

Sedated Strawberries

Serve your dinner liqueur hidden inside a large red strawberry encased in dark chocolate. Yum! This small and perfect dessert idea came from Jane Bailey, a British Columbia cooking teacher and caterer.

PREPARATION TIME: 15 MINUTES / MICROWAVING TIME: 3 MINUTES
REFRIGERATION TIME: 10 MINUTES / MAKES: 12 BERRIES

12 large firm strawberries

2 squares (2 oz/56 g) semisweet or bittersweet chocolate

2 to 3 tbsp orange-flavored liqueur

1. Line a small baking sheet with waxed paper. Leave green hulls on strawberries. Wash berries under cold running water. Pat dry with paper towels.

2. Coarsely chop chocolate and put it in a small microwave-safe dish. Microwave, uncovered, on medium until it is almost melted, about 2 to 3 minutes. Stir until smooth. Or place chopped chocolate into a very small saucepan. Set it over low heat, stirring frequently until melted and smooth, about 5 minutes.

3. Use a plastic syringe to fill berries with liqueur. Fill syringe with some liqueur, then carefully insert needle into hull end of each strawberry. Inject liqueur into center. Refill syringe as needed. Dip end of each berry into chocolate, swirling so chocolate covers about half of berry. Place each berry onto a waxed-paper–lined baking sheet after it is dipped in chocolate. Refrigerate, uncovered, until set, at least 10 minutes. Berries will keep well, refrigerated, for up to half a day. After that time, berries will soften.

SYRINGELESS SEDATED BERRIES: *Pour liqueur over chopped chocolate. Microwave, uncovered, on medium for 2 to 3 minutes. Stir until combined. Mixture will be thick. Using a small spoon or knife, "frost" ends of strawberries with warm chocolate mixture. Place each berry on waxed-paper–lined baking sheet. Refrigerate, uncovered, until set, about 10 minutes.*

PETITE BLUEBERRY CRISP

Stir ¼ cup brown sugar with 1 tablespoon cornstarch until evenly blended. Stir mixture with 2 cups fresh or frozen blueberries in a 6-cup (1.5-L) microwave-safe dish, about 8 inches wide. Cook, uncovered on high, for 4 minutes for fresh berries or 6 minutes for frozen, stirring once, until thick and bubbling. Meanwhile, combine ¼ cup each of all-purpose flour, brown sugar and quick-cooking (but not instant) rolled oats and 2 tablespoons room-temperature butter. Rub mixture together with your fingers until well mixed and crumbly. Spread evenly in a pie plate. Microwave, uncovered, on high 4 minutes, stirring once, until lightly golden and crumbly. Spoon over hot blueberry filling. *Serves 2 to 3.*

PER COATED BERRY

Calories:	41
Protein:	Trace
Fat:	2 g
Carbohydrate:	5 g
Fiber:	1 g

Ultimate Summer Fruit Salad

A hint of ginger perks up melons and berries. This is a gorgeous salad to serve at the end of a barbecue or at a brunch. It's a case of feasting your eyes but not your waistline. For extra glamour, spoon fruit into store-bought meringues and drizzle with a little sour cream or yogurt cheese.

PREPARATION TIME: 15 MINUTES / CHILLING TIME: 3 HOURS
MAKES: 10 ONE-CUP SERVINGS

1 large ripe cantaloupe
1 small honeydew melon (optional)
½ small watermelon
1 pint (500 mL) blueberries
1 pint (500 mL) raspberries or strawberries
1 orange
2 tbsp granulated sugar
¼ cup finely chopped candied ginger

1. Peel, seed and cut melons into 1-inch pieces. Place them in a large bowl and stir in berries. (If using raspberries, add just before serving to avoid mushiness.) Grate peel from orange and squeeze out juice. Stir peel with juice and pour over fruit. Sprinkle salad with sugar and ginger and fold in. Cover and refrigerate until chilled, about 3 hours, or for up to 12 hours before serving.

MINT 'N' HONEY

Stir 1 cup yogurt with 2 tablespoons chopped fresh mint and a squeeze of lemon juice. Stir in 2 tablespoons honey. Taste and add more honey and mint, if you wish. Spoon over fruit salad or berries. *Makes 1¼ cups.*

CITRUS C

Citrus fruits (oranges, grapefruit, lemons and limes) provide an excellent source of vitamin C in our diets. Citrus fruits contain several constituents that, along with the acids in the fruit, prevent the oxidation and loss of vitamin C. Fresh citrus fruits are commonly eaten raw, an added bonus since cooking or heating decreases their nutrient value.

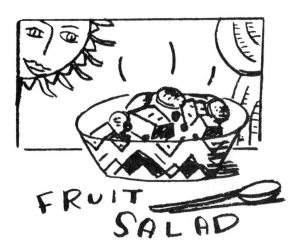

FRUIT SALAD

PER SERVING	
Calories: 119	
Protein: 2 g	
Fat: 1 g	
Carbohydrate: 29 g	
Fiber: 3 g	
Excellent source: Vitamin A, Vitamin C	

A NUTRITIONAL COMPARISON

Type	Calories	Protein (g)	Fat (g)	Carbohydrate (g)
APPLES (1 medium, raw)	82	0	1	21
APRICOTS (10 halves, dried)	83	1	0	22
ASPARAGUS (6 spears, cooked)	20	2	0	4
BROCCOLI (1 cup, cooked)	44	5	1	8
BRUSSELS SPROUTS (1 cup, cooked)	61	4	1	14
CABBAGE (1 cup, raw shredded)	17	1	0	4
CANTALOUPE (1 half)	93	2	1	22
CARROTS (1 medium, raw)	35	1	0	8
CAULIFLOWER (1 cup, raw pieces)	24	2	0	5
MANGOES (1 medium)	135	1	1	35
ORANGES (1 medium)	62	1	0	15
PAPAYA (1 medium)	122	2	0	31
PEPPERS, GREEN (1 raw)	32	1	0	8
PEPPERS, RED (1 raw)	32	1	0	8
POTATOES (1 medium, boiled and peeled)	119	3	0	28
PUMPKIN (1 cup, cooked)	83	3	1	20
RASPBERRIES (1 cup, raw)	60	1	1	14
SPINACH (1 cup, raw)	12	2	0	2
SQUASH, ACORN (¼ medium, baked)	44	1	0	11
STRAWBERRIES (1 cup, raw)	45	1	1	10
SWEET POTATOES (1 medium, baked and peeled)	117	2	0	28
TOMATOES (1 medium, raw)	26	1	0	6

Fiber (g)	Vitamin A (RE)	Vitamin C (mg)	Folic Acid (mcg)	Iron (mg)	Calcium (mg)
3	7	8	4	.2	10
3	253	1	4	1.6	16
1	45	9	122	.6	17
4	217	116	78	1.3	72
7	112	97	94	1.9	56
1	9	33	40	.4	33
2	859	113	45	.6	29
2	2271	8	11	.4	22
2	2	72	66	.6	29
4	806	57	6	.3	21
2	28	70	40	.1	52
5	626	193	3	.3	75
2	75	107	26	.5	11
2	680	227	26	.5	11
2	0	18	14	.4	7
4	4844	9	24	3.4	63
6	16	31	32	.7	27
1	378	16	109	1.5	56
3	34	9	15	.7	35
3	4	85	26	.6	21
3	2484	28	26	.5	32
1	76	23	18	.6	6

Index